TESTIMONIALS OF HEALING

"Per my ENT doctor I have had a constant sinus infection, allergies, or whatever other words he could throw at it for the last year and a half. YES . . . 18 full months of antibiotics, nasal sprays, creams, SURGERY, more sprays, creams, and weeks and weeks of 2 allergy shots per week. Every Day I felt like I drank 3 bottles of wine the night before with no relief. Constant sinus pressure and headaches every single day. I missed 2 summers of swimming with my small kids, trips to the park, and many other fun activities because I simply did not want to move.

I made an appointment with Dr. Segarra, and he told me there was a high probability that my neck was intertwined with the sinus pressures and headaches.

He has me on a 6-8 week plan and right out the gate I am feeling 95% better!!!! Yes . . . there is more work to be done, but I can finally see the light at the end of the tunnel. I can't thank Dr. Segarra and his team enough for what they have done for me."

–CAMERON M.

"I walked in with pain in my knee and was treated like a Rockstar and I walked out with much less pain from the procedure and I was educated on how the knee works."

–JEFFREY BARTLETT

"In the past, he has helped me with my migraines and neck pain. Recently, I was driving and traveling out of town walking a lot more. My lower leg, ankle & foot hurt all of the time, especially trying to sleep. I couldn't walk for exercise and dance with my senior group any longer. I was diagnosed with Neuropathy. I was skeptical in trying Dr. Segarra's treatment that included laser, infrared, LED light, microcurrent, vibration & muscle treatment techniques. After a few treatments I noticed I was sleeping and walking better. I resumed my regular activities. His team will greet you with a smile and always make you feel welcome. It has been a blessing working with them."

—BECKY BARNES

"I really do not know what I would do if I had not found Dr. Segarra. I was in severe pain 24 hours a day and could not move my body without help from my husband. I could hardly walk upon arrival at his office. I was using a cane and had a previous diagnosis of neuropathy. I was glad that the evaluation included X-rays and consultation. He had a plan for me to be dancing by December for my 50th wedding anniversary. This was in October. I was indeed dancing in December. Not only that but guess what, neuropathy is not a problem and I have avoided knee replacement and my sciatica is gone. I am able to continue my traveling with my husband and move without assistance. Office staff is wonderful also. Thanks to all of you."

—ELIZABETH ORR

"I have rheumatoid arthritis and since I've started coming here I've noticed such a decrease in pain and flare ups."

—JESSICA WIKE

"Dr. Segarra and his staff are excellent and have helped me over-
come and improve multiple problems from leg pain, lower back
pain, neck pain, rotator cuff locking, and shoulder pain. Recently
I developed tinnitus and it has greatly improved with just a few
treatments. The adjustments and therapy treatments really work,
along with the exercises they encourage you to do with each
different problem. Their treatments keep me going and enjoying
life in my senior years! "

–ANN WALTERS

"About 9 weeks ago I hurt my back and was worried that I
would need surgery to repair it. My mom had suggested I go
to Harrisburg Wellness Center. So I did. On my initial visit I
was very nervous that a Chiropractor could not help me. Boy
was I wrong. Dr. Segarra informed me I had herniated my L4
disk which was leading to severe sciatica issues in my left leg
that went all the way to my toes tingling. He told me it could be
repaired with a comprehensive therapy program. So the process
started with decompression and Laser therapy. He found the
spot in the nerve that was causing me so much pain. Thanks to
Dr. Segarra and his staff, doing decompression and Laser Therapy, 9 weeks later I am back 90% of my strength without having
to have surgery and on my way back to 100%. I would definitely
recommend their services."

–CHRIS ALMOND

"Tingling and numbness in my feet are gone from diabetic neuropathy. My balance, standing and walking are so much better."

–MANUAL SAN JOSE

"Dr. Segarra was simply the best thing to ever happen to our family! My daughter was in a car accident and after seeing many medical specialists, no one could figure out how to treat her consistent and extremely painful headaches. After the very first treatment, her headaches were drastically reduced and with her continued care, she is headache and head pain free! My husband also suffers with flexibility issues from deployments to Iraq & Afghanistan. Care from Dr. Segarra has been a total game changer! I was very skeptical of chiropractic care and I now see how foolish that was. No more pain pills in this house! We truly appreciate Dr. Segarra and his staff!!"

—JENNIFER POOL

"I have struggled with headaches/migraines my whole life and bad back/neck pain with my four pregnancies. After one week seeing Dr. Segarra I can already see a noticeable difference in my pain, and am able to pick up my toddler without any pain. I am able to move and turn my neck much easier and haven't had a single headache. From the start, I have had a great experience with Dr. Segarra and his staff. The most important thing to me though, is every time I walk in the door, everyone has a smile on their face and they are just so friendly and uplifting. I always leave in a better mood than when I arrived."

—ASHLEY HALL

"My neuropathy in my feet that felt like burning, cold sensation and walking on tacks is doing so much better. I am playing golf again, walking normally and even running. Come see Dr. Segarra. It's worth your time."

—MATT LIPOMI

"I have been seeing Dr. Segarra for 5 weeks for my knees and foot problems. I was in extreme pain. Now I am practically out of pain. I am walking, sleeping and exercising better. I have to travel one way 35 minutes to get to his office, but he is well worth it. He told me I may have an autoimmune disease and I should have my blood work done. I did and I do. I am doing things to reduce my levels of inflammation."

–LUCY STEPHAN

"Dr. Segarra has done some really great work on my shoulder. When I thought I had a rotator cuff issue and required surgery, he was able to work the extremity with a number of movements and treatment. I play tennis regularly and the shoulder has zero pain. A great alternative to surgery! Highly recommend him for sports related injuries."

–PAUL DRAKE

"Plantar Fasciitis - I was suffering with plantar fasciitis for about a month. Whenever I walked, any pressure on my left heel was painful and caused me to limp. I love to play pickleball, but I couldn't and I missed it a LOT. On a recent trip to Charlotte NC I visited Dr. Segarra. He provided soft tissue treatments, stretching, laser treatments and gave me a regiment for icing and exercises I could do on my own. Within a week, after only two treatments, the pain was gone and I'm back playing Pickleball. WOW - What a GREAT result. . . . I'd recommend him to anyone after this!!!!"

–ROBERT WELD

"I highly recommend Dr. Segarra and his staff. Paige and Mindy are wonderful and make you feel like family. You can tell they care and will go the extra mile to help you.

Dr. Segarra is very knowledgeable and experienced and will go over and above to help you. I went there out of desperation to alleviate my neuropathy symptoms and the treatment regimen definitely helped. If you have neuropathy, go see them at least for the initial exam. It is very thorough and he will explain the tests in as much detail as you want. There is no pressure at all. He will explain the proposed treatment plan and the rest is up to you.

Again, I highly recommend them and have to say again that Paige and Mindy are absolutely wonderful! I don't want to be in pain again but if I am I know where I will go!"

–RC ALLEN

"As a software developer, I sit in a chair for long stretches of time. Consequently, this caused chronic neck and lower back pain. I went to Dr. Segarra and he has been highly effective in treating these conditions. I'm now able to hold my head straight ahead while reading or looking at a computer screen.

He is a very caring doctor. He spends considerable time learning about my activities so that he can provide the best treatment. He also spends adequate time with me in the Exam Room. On one occasion I suffered from vertigo - the whole room was spinning. Worst thing I ever experienced! I went to Dr. Segarra and with his treatments it solved the problem and I have not had vertigo ever since. He is meticulous, caring, and diligent. I highly recommend him."

–GINGER DAY

"If you are getting serious about your health, you should check out Dr. Segarra's wellness center (aka. Harrisburg Chiropractic). He takes a whole body approach to supporting you to improve your health. My family and I appreciate that Dr. Segarra and his team took time to gather all of the health related concerns and goals. Then they came up with a plan, explained options and techniques. As new concerns have come up, they have adjusted treatment techniques and scheduling as needed. If you are not getting what you need from your current chiropractor, you may want to check out Dr. Segarra for a more complete care approach."

—DAVID KOHLER

"I came to Dr. Segarra with over 8 years of lower back pain and leg numbness. Between his high energy and smooth consultation I knew relief was on the way. Based on my x-rays he knew what was causing my issue. We agreed on a treatment plan and went to work. After 2 weeks of therapy I'm happy to say that I am sleeping soundly to my alarm for a change. Did I mention that I've had 2 weeks of back pain free, numb legs free work week? I'm now able to play in the yard with my younger grandchildren and shoot basketball with the older grandsons. Thank you for giving me my life back . . . My future looks a lot brighter with no pain."

—REGGIE BROWN

"I started seeing Dr. Segarra for fatigue, extreme migraine headaches and gut issues. I was seeing a neurologist and using a heart monitor. I am now able to care for my 3 kids again, I'm back driving to work and working as a hairdresser again. Thanks Dr. Segarra! "

-AVA QUICK

"I came in after a bad reaction to a statin drug and arthritic issues, unable to walk well or straighten out my right leg. I was told I would need a knee replacement. Ortho doc gave up on me, my knee and sciatica but Dr. Segarra did not. After three treatments I was straightening out my leg and walking better. He also fixed old injuries that were activated by the reaction to the drug. I am spring cleaning and walking around the mall again. He is dedicated to his patients. Thank You for helping me get my life back Dr. Segarra."

-JUDY PEPPER

"I was having severe hip problems and pain. Orthopedic doctor stated I needed a hip replacement. I thought since I can exercise and dance why would I need a hip replacement, so I tried Harrisburg Chiropractic and I gradually noticed the pain and stiffness was disappearing. 12 sessions and the pain is completely gone. Apparently I did not need a hip replacement. Thank you Dr. Segarra. And, I thought this would not help but was willing to try anything."

-CAROLYN REESE

"Bone on bone knee arthritis. My orthopedist gave me cortisone shots in both knees. He said I needed knee replacements. Wake Forest then gave me lubrication shots with little improvement. I was constantly taking over the counter meds. I'm now able to walk and stand so much better, sleeping great and finally walking up and down stairs again. I'm keeping up with my grandkids again."

–JACK BRANSCOME

"20 years of neuropathy in my feet and hands while taking Gabapentin. Playing golf, walking more confidently again after losing my balance and falling in the past. I can actually feel the tees in my pocket again and can button my shirt. Started dancing with my wife again. Thanks Dr. Segarra."

– HOUSTON LEIGH

"20 + years of arthritic knee pain. I have tried cortisone, gel, serum injections with no help. I am a cyclist and am now back to biking 5 to 7 hours at a time with no pain. I feel like I've turned back the clock 30 years. You need to come in and see what the good doctor can do for you as well."

–CURTIS HENDERSON

BREAKTHROUGH
TO
HEALING

BREAKTHROUGH TO HEALING

CONNECTING ROOT CAUSES OF
CHRONIC HEALTH CONDITIONS
WITH ALTERNATIVE SOLUTIONS

DR. ANDREW SEGARRA, DC, CCEP, AFNI-C

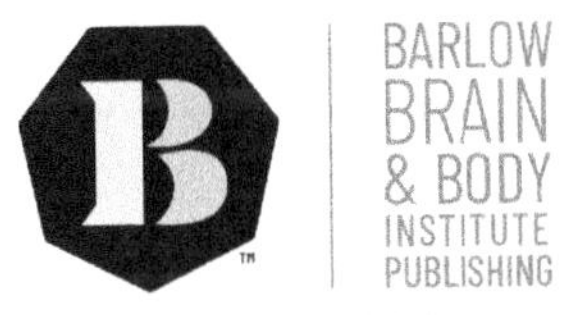

BARLOW BRAIN & BODY INSTITUTE PUBLISHING

Thank you:

Early on in my career, when it appeared that the windows of opportunity were closing for me, I was fortunate enough to meet Dr. Steve Binder, Dr. Bob Stroud and the late Dr. Mike Binder. They gave me an opportunity I had always hoped for: to run and eventually own my own clinic. I am forever grateful. Dr. Ed Reilly walked into my life during another transition in my career. His friendship, support and guidance has been instrumental in the level of care we offer. It is a constant pursuit and evolution to improve patient care and offer the latest in regenerative treatments. Thank you for this journey.

It is never easy being an entrepreneur. There are always trials and tribulations when you own your own business. My wife's kindness, patience and unconditional love and support are just a few of the attributes that have helped me through all of the challenges. The sacrifices you have made for me and our family never go unnoticed. Thank you for all you have done and continue to do. You truly have and continue to make me a better person.

TABLE OF CONTENTS

FOREWORD

As a physician, I see so many patients suffering from chronic disease. And along with the disease often come many questions from patients. How did this happen? What could I have done to avoid it? Will I get better? What do I do now?

What if we had the know-how and ability to cut some diseases off before they even had a chance to get a foothold on our health? I believe the information inside this book answers many of those questions and is so powerful that it will likely forever change our clinical perspectives on the importance of maintaining a healthy physiological state within our bodies.

Breakthrough to Healing – Connecting Root Causes of Chronic Health Conditions with Alternative Solutions might be considered the "owner's manual" for fighting, beating and even preventing disease. The practical steps and inside-out approach Dr. Segarra discusses in this book helps you envision a battle plan to beat even the most chronic conditions.

Dr. Segarra keys in on so many facts and simple ways to think about your health. The information he presents in this book holds some important methodologies to finding and mastering control of your well-being.

This entire book, page by page, could profoundly impact the way you view healthcare and give you the hope and tools to prevent and fight the ever-increasing diagnosis of chronic disease. As you pour through the information, you will surely find it fascinating, inspiring, and even the topic of daily conversation and practical use.

No one is immune to the onset of disease. However, when we are armed with the right information, we have a fighting chance to fend off the perils of chronic illness and pain. *Breakthrough to Healing – Connecting Root Causes of Chronic Health Conditions with Alternative Solutions* offers the jewels of knowledge and the direction we need. As such, this book is surely destined to become legendary and Dr. Segarra is a hero for his patients and anyone who reads this book. Thank you Dr. Segarra for bringing this information to light for the world to embrace.

Dr. Michael Perusich, BS, MS, DC, LMn, DICCP, FICC

PART ONE

SHARED PHILOSOPHY

CHAPTER 1

A DIFFERENT KIND OF DOCTOR

was first introduced to chiropractic when I fell off my neighbor's garage roof as a 5-year-old and injured my back. My mom had been going to a chiropractor for her chronic health issues, so it was an easy decision for her to take me there for help. The two of us would utilize chiropractic throughout my upbringing. At the same time, my dad would always say to me, "Go out and own your own business. Don't work in a corporate setting like me, there's too much bureaucracy to deal with." He did the books for my dentist for a few years and knew I enjoyed science and math so he'd encourage me to do something along those lines. I went on to study biology and athletic training in college. All things considered, being able to help people by becoming a chiropractor became very appealing to me.

Despite that, I had my reservations back then. Chiropractic wasn't and still isn't "mainstream" healthcare. There were a lot of misconceptions about the profession that I bought into and many people still do today. I didn't really understand what it was all about. But when I graduated in 1998 and started treating people, I began to see how big of an impact I was having in helping people. I knew the road would have challenges, but I now had some confidence, a new calling, and a purpose in my life.

I guess you could say that I'm not your stereotypical "rack 'em and crack 'em" kind of chiropractor. I decided to attend a chiropractic school that taught me more ways than just chiropractic adjusting to help people. At the National University of Health Sciences in Lumbard, IL I was able to learn from multiple disciplines including acupuncture and nutrition. I became a sponge learning many ways to help people without drugs or surgery.

I had a rehab professor who taught me about exercise, strengthening, stretching, and all things related to physical therapy. That was pretty unheard of to see a physical therapist in a chiropractic school back then. I looked at learning from someone who sees healthcare from a different vantage point other than chiropractic as a benefit.

With the school's connections, I was selected for a hospital rotation program. I knew my education had been training me to be a more "natural" primary care physician but didn't fully realize the extent of my knowledge until I got to observe surgeries and go on rounds with the medical residents. We'd discuss each hospitalized patient's condition, the reason for ordering tests and their results in coming up with a proper diagnosis. It gave me the confidence and understanding that I had the tools to properly diagnose complex patient health conditions and discuss them in detail with medical practitioners. The difference would be in how I would treat those ailments in a more natural way with far fewer side effects than drugs or surgery.

When it came time to study for the board exams, I always felt like I had an advantage due to all of the hands-on experience I got from my time in the hospital. It made me feel like it was harder on students in other chiropractic schools who didn't have those kinds of experiences and had to go back and study and help each other recall information before the test. It was much fresher in my mind and easier to recall because I lived it.

After working on hospital rotations for a while, I got accepted into an AIDS alternative health project. Back then, people were dying from AIDS. I had the opportunity to learn the phases and treatment plans behind the disease I was hearing so much about on the news. Patients were on aggressive "medical cocktails," and I was there working on alternative methods to help them. It was challenging as patients were passing away. I appreciated that my school exposed me to so many different healthcare settings and difficult health conditions. Having these experiences helped open my mind to the idea that helping people with complex chronic illnesses from a natural standpoint would become a new calling for me later in practice.

After graduation, I worked in a multi-disciplinary clinic that was set up with an urgent care facility. I got to work with different medical doctors who were on staff with me. We saw many different patient ailments. If there were any muscle, joint or nerve issues, they'd be directed to those of us who were chiropractors and physical therapists. We had a large rehabilitative gym area for treatments. On days when we were short-staffed, I'd help by setting up outpatients for the medical doctors to see.

This clinic enabled me to get to know some of the MD's well. We'd collaborate on lab tests and x-rays and through many conversations, I got to see and understand their rationale and decision making in treating patients.

I recall one MD I worked with said he enjoyed working at our clinic because he never had to prescribe powerful, addictive pain medications that patients may abuse. He would simply refer them to the chiropractic and physical therapy side of our clinic for treatment.

Taking in all that I'd learned from hospital rounds and surgeries, the AIDS alternative health project, and having worked at a multi-disciplinary clinic with medical doctors and physical therapists helped open me up to referral networks and collaboration with other healthcare disciplines in treating patients that I still utilize today.

I began practicing on my own in 2001, just outside of Charlotte, North Carolina. I recognized most patients go to a medical doctor as the first point of contact for any ailment. I wanted to reach a larger audience that could benefit from my services. There were so many misconceptions about how I practiced that I felt I needed to bridge that gap. I was able to lean on my past experiences working alongside the medical community, presented research articles and demonstrated equipment I utilized in patient care by arranging meetings at local medical clinics. I wasn't going to sit back and hope potential patients would see my sign out in front of my clinic and expect that my practice would take off. That's not how it works in my profession. You have to reach out to the community and start establishing relationships. To this day, I still work hard to develop connections and referral networks with many businesses, organizations and groups in our area. The medical community was and still is one of those relationships. If I didn't reach out, so many patients in my area would never benefit from the services I have to offer. If a patient asks and/or consents for us to keep their MD in the loop on their treatment with us, I am always happy to oblige with the patient's progress notes. It's all about establishing relationships for the betterment of patient care and patient outcomes.

CHAPTER 2

THE IDEAS THAT COMPEL ME

've seen the power of finding a path that leads to long-term healing for people. It's important for me to share what I've learned with prospective and current patients to help break down some of the stereotypes and myths about my diagnosis and treatment methodology and educate people on the benefits with real examples from my first-hand experiences. That being said, I'd like to share my core beliefs as a health care practitioner and why working with me can be beneficial to anyone looking for a better path to true healing.

IT'S ABOUT THE QUALITY OF YOUR LIFE

What are the things that you can't do right now that you want to be able to do again? Are you as productive as you once were performing work activities? Are you sleeping soundly through the night? Can you get out of bed or up and down stairs without difficulty? Are you able to travel and perform exercise or recreational activities without discomfort? Is it getting harder to landscape your home or take care of your household? Are you concerned you won't be able to live independently in your home for the rest of your life? Will friends or family members have to step in to care for you as you age?

You need to ask yourself: if I keep doing what I have been doing to address my health issues, what will my lifestyle look like in three, five or ten years? Will I be better or worse off? Am I struggling, thinking my health can't get any better? Is it time to address my problems from a different perspective?

If you don't like what you see, the only person who can make significant changes is you. With the right information, you can make the changes that alter the course of your health for the better.

PERPETUAL MEDICATION USE IS NOT HEALTHY FOR PEOPLE WITH CHRONIC HEALTH ISSUES

For patients with long-term health challenges, taking medications for the remainder of their life isn't necessarily getting them healthy. To me, medicine was invented to help your symptoms (the end result of your problem) and help get things under control until you make the necessary lifestyle changes that caused the problem in the first place. It's a common misconception that too many people buy into. The fact of the matter is that you aren't meant to be on the same medications for the rest of your life. You may find yourself in that position because you are realizing that you never actually treated the main cause of the health problem you're dealing with.

Contrary to the way pharmaceutical companies market their products to us, there is no magic pill that will solve your health challenges overnight. What people don't realize is that when you take one medication for a specific condition, very often it will help the symptoms associated with that condition. If you must continuously take that medication, you may not be addressing the condition's root cause. Instead, you are merely managing the condition's symptoms (or at least the symptoms that are displaying themselves) to some extent while it can cause new problems. Then you are prescribed a second medication to combat the side effects from the first one. It's a cascading effect that too many of my patients with complex, chronic health issues had no idea what they were signing up for. By the time someone decides to see me, they've been on five, sometimes twenty medications for multiple years that have only combated their symptoms, never addressing the causes as their overall health continues to deteriorate.

TAKING OWNERSHIP OF YOUR HEALTH IS KEY TO YOUR SUCCESS

When you work with a chiropractor, it is important that you understand you are creating a partnership within a learning environment. Keep an open mind and know that action is required on your part to take in new information and implement what you've learned into your daily life.

You didn't get where you are today overnight, and you can't expect to obtain a cure after one appointment. But when you choose to work with someone like me that will develop a plan of attack, you'll begin to understand the root causes of the health problems you're dealing with and how to truly get on a path to healing. It takes time but can lead to ending or reversing the course of a particular health condition. You may even be able to ditch all those prescribed medications over time as you step away from the traditional way of treating symptoms.

LEARNING ABOUT YOUR BODY IS THE BEST WAY TO TAKE CARE OF IT

My favorite part of being a chiropractor is having the privilege of taking the wisdom I've gained over the years and using it to educate others. I've always felt compelled to give people the why behind the what when we create a treatment plan. In fact, that is exactly why we're here together right now. In the following chapters, I'd like to provide you with user-friendly information on your body's systems and how to best take care of them. Let the learning begin!

CHAPTER 3

THERE'S MORE BELOW THE SURFACE

TIP OF THE ICEBERG

Have you ever studied a diagram of an iceberg? From above the surface of the water, your eye can only see about 10% of the iceberg's total mass while the remaining 90% remains out of sight, lurking below the surface. An iceberg is a good metaphor for the way we should understand the total picture of our health. The symptoms we experience represent only 10-15% of the issue that is causing those obvious symptoms to appear. To understand the whole picture, uncover the web of dysfunction, and discover the path to true healing, we have to delve below the surface.

Symptoms can also be compared to the check engine light on your car. If you're on a road trip and the check engine light comes on, you're alerted to a problem with your vehicle. Would taking a piece of duct tape and covering up that check engine light solve the problem? Absolutely not, it would only prevent you from seeing the blinking light that's alerting you to a bigger issue. In fact, covering up the check engine light puts you in greater danger in the long run because what started out as a small problem will get worse and worse if you continue on your road trip and don't address the problem. Pretty soon, you're sitting on the side of the road with smoke and steam rolling out of your engine. This is what it's like when we take medication to mask our symptoms. Covering them up doesn't change the fact that there's a problem. To really figure out the issue with our car, we must go to a mechanic and have them look under the hood. To figure out the issue with our body, we need to untangle the web of dysfunction that's causing the symptom to surface.

In a car, there are a multitude of reasons why the check engine light appears. It could be a fuel issue, a spark plug issue, a battery issue, or something else entirely. Think of your health symptoms as your body's check engine light. In the same way that a check engine light comes on for a variety of reasons, our symptoms can result from a variety of health issues. This is one of the most important concepts that I teach my patients - the root cause of symptoms is different for every single person because their web of dysfunction is completely unique.

There are three main reasons why a "one size fits all" strategy does not work for solving chronic health problems. The first reason is that two people could be experiencing the same exact symptoms for completely different reasons. For example, numbness, tingling or burning of the feet can be caused by nerve damage in the lumbar spine at the L5 vertebrae. However, it can also be caused by Type 2 diabetes or anemia. All three disorders can cause the exact same symptom for totally different reasons. To make the tangled web of dysfunction even more complicated, many of my patients have more than one root cause of their symptoms. The bottom line is that every person's health issues must be treated uniquely.

The second reason why a "one size fits all" approach doesn't work is because a doctor with preconceived notions tends to miss important clues that reveal what's really going on beneath the surface. For someone with chronic health problems, there are multiple mechanisms that can go awry and cause dysfunction, yet show up as the same kind of symptom. These mechanisms include elements like blood sugar, anemia, or destruction of the neurological pathways. If the root cause is never addressed, the correct mechanism that needs restoration and healing will never be found. Each person is a custom case. As a functional neuro-metabolic doctor, it's my job to be smart enough to look below the surface and examine the 90% that's beneath the surface.

The third reason why a "one size fits all approach" does not work for solving chronic health problems is because it tends to produce doctors that are symptom-reduction oriented rather than results oriented. As a functional neuro-medicine doctor, I want my patients to actually get better. Every time I walk into a room with a patient, I check my ego at the door because I want to solve their problems, not mask them. I am result oriented, and I am solution oriented. I'm committed to getting results for my patients, and I will exhaust all of my resources to do it. I treat each patient like a custom, one-of-a-kind 10,000 piece puzzle. When I accept a patient for care, we sit down together and start working on that puzzle until we uncover the root cause(s) and form a plan to heal them. To truly heal, we need to target and solve the core problem. We must untangle the neuro-metabolic web of dysfunction and start a journey to regeneration and wellness.

With the first three chapters as our foundation, let's go deeper by defining and then explaining the Seven Keys to healing your chronic health problems.

PART TWO

SHARED UNDERSTANDING

CHAPTER 4

UNTANGLING THE WEB OF DYSFUNCTION

There are seven key areas of health that I look at when I'm trying to untangle someone's web of dysfunction. Depending on
how they're treated, these seven keys can either foster wellness
and longevity or create debilitating chronic health problems
because each of these keys either adds to our health or active-
ly takes away and destroys our health. Throughout my years of
practice and study, I've discovered that any kind of disruption
in these seven areas is going to cause disconnection and dysfunction (check engine light) which may eventually turn into
chronic issues. When I work with a patient to help them with
their chronic health problems, this is always where we begin.
When these seven areas are treated well, it unleashes your body's
superpower which is its ability to heal itself.

THE SEVEN KEYS

1. Oxygen: Number One of the BIG Three. It is necessary
    and essential for life. Anoxia (which means "without ox-
    ygen") equals death. The brain and nervous system need
    three elements to function at peak level, and oxygen is
    one of them. Oxygen is the deal breaker when it comes
    to neurological health. The less oxygen we have in our

bodies, the more things start to malfunction and the less capacity our bodies have to heal themselves.

2. Glucose: Number Two of the BIG Three. Glucose is your blood sugar. It's the fuel that your body needs in order to heal itself. It's also needed for the nervous system to self-regulate and function optimally. A good metaphor is that it's like the gasoline for your car engine. Cars run at a certain octane level, and if that level gets out of balance, the car isn't going to run properly. Our bodies work the same way with glucose. If there's too little, it can't function at its optimal level. If there's too much, it's not good for optimal performance either.

3. Stimulation: Number Three of the BIG Three. Stimulation is one of the main three things that the nervous system needs in order to function. The importance of stimulation can't be overstated. As Einstein once said, "Nothing happens until something moves," and in the body, no healing happens until something is stimulated. Without stimulation, the body's systems will weaken and fail. With proper stimulation, those systems will thrive and remain strong.

4. Autoimmune Disorders: Autoimmune disorders are kind of like "friendly fire." They develop when our immune system starts attacking itself instead of a foreign invader. Our immune systems should only kill the "bad guys" like viruses, but when it starts to malfunction, it doesn't just destroy antigens, it also attacks our own tissues.

5. Inflammation: Logic tells you that if your house was on fire, you wouldn't start rebuilding it until after the blazes were put out. Inflammation is like a fire in your body, and it can't start to heal until that fire is gone. True healing cannot take place until your body's inflammation is reduced.

6. Neurotoxins: These toxins are anything that's taken into the body that causes neurological damage. Unfortunately neurotoxins are much more common than you may imagine. Table sugar is a neurotoxin. High fructose corn syrup is a neurotoxin. The artificial sweeteners Aspartame (NutraSweet), and Sucralose (Splenda) are neurotoxins. Drinking water out of a disposable plastic bottle is neurotoxic. We'll talk more in upcoming chapters about how to eliminate these harmful toxins from your life.

7. Gut Health: The role of gut health is paramount because poor gut health is a trigger for autoimmune conditions and out of control inflammatory responses. We must heal our guts in order to heal our brains and bodies. If you have a bad brain, you're guaranteed to have a bad gut too. We must restore optimal gut health and reconnect the gut-brain axis in order to achieve true healing.

While each of these seven areas are important to address individually, their true power for healing comes alive when we realize that all of these elements are interconnected. Gut health and autoimmune conditions are connected. Neurotoxins and inflammation are linked. Oxygen and stimulation are crucial to one another's roles. The body is a holistic system that must be in homeostasis in order to heal itself and function optimally. By keeping these seven primary keys in focus, your health can transform from symptom mitigation to a state of true healing and regeneration. Now that we've looked at an overview of the seven keys to optimal health, let's break each key down in greater detail.

CHAPTER 5

KEY 1 – OXYGEN

THE ROLE OF OXYGEN

Oxygen is essential for life. This element, which makes up about 21% of the earth's atmosphere at sea level, is key to our health because our bodies need it in order to function on a cellular level. We can go without food almost forty days, and we can last about four days without water. However, we can only survive for approximately four minutes without oxygen. If the brain is deprived of oxygen for longer than that, it's a recipe for severe neurological damage and even death. Our cells need oxygen in order to make ATP, which is essentially the "energy" on which our bodies run. If there isn't adequate energy, then the neurons (the cells responsible for receiving sensory input from the outside world and for sending motor commands to our muscles) fail and many forms of neurological dysfunction and chronic health problems may follow.

Oxygen deprivation isn't only a reality for people who need to be "on oxygen" or are constantly hooked up to a machine. In fact, I see many, many patients who are lacking oxygen because they're anemic. An anemic person may have decreased blood circulation issues which equals decreased oxygen to the tissues of the body. Many of my patients have been anemic for years but no doctor has taken the time to explain to them what that means for their health so they don't understand the full implications of that diagnosis.

Our bodies must have an adequate supply of oxygen in order to heal, especially when it comes to chronic health problems. Oxygen plays a crucial role in helping us heal from chronic health issues because of something called "resting membrane potential of the nerve cells." When a nerve is asked to perform a task but it's lacking oxygen, it's similar to an empty soap dispenser. You can pump and pump but nothing is going to happen. On the contrary, when the dispenser is full, it may be so primed that soap is coming out without any pumping. In the same way, oxygen impacts the nervous system's ability to function because it's what "primes the pump" for the nerve cells and gives it the energy to do its job.

The nervous system is made up of individual cells called neurons, and to maintain the health of these neurons, oxygen is crucial. Healthy neurons and an optimally functioning nervous system are essential building blocks for structural integrity of the cells, fighting chronic health issues and healing the body. Let's take a moment to dive deeper into understanding neurons and their function in our bodies.

A neuron's job is to transmit communication from the brain to the body and from the body back to the brain. Neurons communicate in two ways: electronically (similar to the electrical system in your home) and chemically (called neurotransmitters). In order for neurons to optimize communication between the brain and the body (and vice versa), they need three things: oxygen, glucose, and stimulation. If any of one of those three elements are taken away, you get neurons that don't "fire" properly, and malfunctioning neurons may cause brain fog, attention, memory issues as well as numbness, tingling and pins and needles sensation in the body.

If these neurons are interfered with, stunted, blunted or damaged in any way, the stage is set for an environment of dysfunction, which then may lead to a disease process.

To understand the disruptive effect of malfunctioning neurons, consider your home's internet connection. When the connection is interrupted or slowed, problems begin to appear. Your Netflix show appears grainy or your pictures don't download properly. Now think about your brain trying to communicate with all 75 trillion cells in your body. Imagine how easily things could go awry in that kind of system. So it is with our bodies and the complex wonder that is our neurological system. If the neurons that comprise our neurological system don't have an adequate supply of oxygen, the body can't heal itself properly because its main communication system is compromised.

There are a few ways to discover if you are oxygen deficient or not. To test a patient's oxygen levels at the clinic, I use a tool called a pulse oximeter. It's put on the tip of the finger and measures oxygen levels. Another way to test oxygen levels is by taking a person's blood pressure. If it's too low, it means the tissues of the body are not getting enough blood supply, and blood is what transports oxygen within the body. The third way to test oxygen levels is through blood work. I look at the total red blood cell count, and if that's too low, it's a sign of oxygen deficiency. These measurement tools are used to see how oxygen deficient someone may be and helps me determine how to treat them best. Signs of poor circulation are cold hands, cold feet, white fingernails (should be pink in color), and nail fungus. There's a saying in functional neurology, "cold hands, cold feet equals cold brain." Meaning, if you have poor circulation in your hands and feet, you probably have poor circulation in your brain as well.

RESULTS FROM OXYGEN

In order to understand how important oxygen is for healing chronic health problems, the main thing to grasp is that a person's oxygen level determines how much stimulation can be put into their nervous system before it "fails" (aka ceases to properly relay the stimulation). This system failure is known as "exceeding metabolic capacity" or EMC. At that point, the nervous system can take no more stimulation and may react with a headache, dizziness, or equilibrium problems.

If you're suffering from anemia, the first thing you may experience is a lack of concentration, focus, and attention. This may eventually turn into memory loss and dementia, but if you catch it early enough, it may be reversed. Lack of oxygen may also cause your extremities to change color, your nails to turn white, or you may lack hair on your lower extremities.

When your body is deficient of oxygen, many internal systems begin to misfire and go awry. The signals traveling from the body to your brain travel at roughly 268 mph. If there's a lack of oxygen, those major neural pathways become compromised and can't convey those fast-moving signals. If your oxygen level is skewed at all, it can lead to numbness, tingling, sensations of pins and needles, and other strange symptoms that show the neurons are misfiring.

There are a few simple, at-home tests you can do to see if you are anemic, aka lacking oxygen and lack of circulation. Start by looking at your fingernails. Are they pink? (Pink is good.) Or are they white? (White is bad.) What color are your toes? Are they blue? (Blue is bad.) Or purple? (Purple very bad.) You can also check for "pitting edema." If you push your finger into your lower leg and it doesn't rebound quickly, you are likely anemic. Toe fungus is another clue that you're not getting enough oxygen to your extremities, or if you always have cold fingers and toes (or cold extremities in general) that's a sign of anemia and poor circulation.

Bloodwork is also a great way to tell if you're lacking oxygen. If you've had blood tests in the last six months, examine your results to see if your red blood cell (RBC) count is low. If it is, that's a clue. If your hemoglobin (HGB) is too low, you are anemic. If you have low hematocrit (HCT) that's also an indicator of anemia. Your blood is like the 18-wheeler that delivers oxygen to your body's tissues, so those numbers are solid indicators of whether you're getting adequate oxygen supply or not.

If you suspect you are anemic, increasing the supply of oxygen to your body may impact your overall health in many positive ways. First of all, you'll notice an increase in energy and endurance and your mental endurance will also improve. You may also notice a better ability to focus for long periods of time. Many patients tell me they start sleeping better, feel better and have more mental clarity. All of these positive results start to happen because the neurons have enough oxygen to fire properly.

YOUR FIRST STEP

There are many simple ways to increase your oxygen levels. At the clinic, I often have anemic patients do exercise with oxygen therapy. They put an oxygen supply mask over their face while completing a low impact exercise, called Exercise With Oxygen Therapy (EWOT). This is a very powerful therapy for oxygenating the body as well as the brain, because not only is oxygen being pumped through the mask, but the body and brain naturally increase their ability to receive oxygen as well as improve circulation when performing EWOT.

A few other simple strategies to increase oxygen levels include walking for at least thirty minutes per day and doing deep breathing exercises. Deep breathing or "forced breathing" exercises actually help stimulate the frontal lobe areas of your brain. The key to forced breathing is a 1:2 ratio. Start with breathing in deeply for four seconds and out for eight seconds, if you can perform this task move up to six seconds in and twelve seconds out. Optimal performance would be eight seconds in and sixteen seconds out. For chronic health suffers, eight in and sixteen out will be a challenge. These activities cause stimulation to the neurological pathways and inundate the body with oxygen. If you can't currently walk for thirty minutes, start by walking for five or six minutes per day. The most important thing is to stimulate the neurological system. Motion is life! Bicycling, either on a stationary bike or outdoors, is also excellent. Don't forget about swimming, it's low impact on your joints and very beneficial to your health. Take what you have at home and use it. It doesn't cost you anything to go outside and walk or do some forced breathing exercises.

When you go for your daily walk, swing your arms in an over exaggerated fashion. Non-linear complex movements (figure eight motions or writing your A,B,C's) will stimulate your cerebellum which in turn stimulates your brain. It's a win-win because it not only gets blood flowing to the extremity doing the non-linear movement, it also increases blood flow to the part of the cerebellum and brain which controls your extremities.

Now that we've covered the key health element of oxygen, let's look at the next key to improving chronic health problems.

CHAPTER 6

KEY 2 – GLUCOSE

THE ROLE OF GLUCOSE

You may have heard the word "glucose" before, but what exactly is it and why is it so important to our health? Glucose is simply our blood sugar, and it's the "fuel" that drives our nervous system. It plays an essential role in healing chronic problems because it supplies our nervous system with the energy it needs to do its job. Of course, healing only happens when our glucose is in optimal range (85-99) and when our A1C is below 5.3. Both of these numbers are a part of routine bloodwork.

In the same way that a car needs the proper fuel for its engine to start and to drive down the road, your nervous system needs the right levels of glucose to function optimally. Not only is the type of fuel important, the amount of fuel is key as well. If you don't have enough glucose, your body can't create the energy it needs to function. (Anything below 85 is hypoglycemia.) Yet if there's too much glucose present in your body, you'll feel slow, sluggish, and tired after eating. (Anything above 99 is hypergly-cemia.) An abundance of glucose can also have a severely dam-aging effect on the nervous system. The higher the number, the more damaging the effects to your nervous system, brain, blood vessels and organs resulting in problems such as kidney failure or blindness.

There are a few ways to measure the glucose levels of your body. The first and most common way is through a simple blood test. Based on your results, you can see if your glucose (aka blood sugar) levels are too high or too low. The most simple, inexpensive (free!) at-home "test" to evaluate your glucose levels is to pay attention to the way you feel before and after meals.

If your blood sugar is too low (a condition known as "hypoglycemia"), you will feel a lack of concentration and focus as well as irritability prior to eating. Have you ever heard the term "hangry?" After you eat and your body becomes inundated with glucose, you'll start to feel better. If your glucose levels are too low, you may also have a tendency to wake up at night, have trouble sleeping, and often skip breakfast.

If your glucose levels are too high (known as "hyperglycemia"), you'll likely feel sleepy and sluggish after eating, especially if your meal contains lots of carbohydrates. Too much blood sugar may also cause you to be constantly thirsty, have headaches, or have trouble concentrating.

When your glucose levels are properly balanced, you don't experience the "hangry" feelings, the "crash" after a meal, or the constant cravings for sugars and starches. The only thing that should happen after you eat is that you feel full. That's it.

RESULTS FROM GLUCOSE

Let's dive deeper into what happens when you have a deficiency of glucose. The first symptoms of low blood sugar are the loss of focus, concentration, and attention. Many hypoglycemic people experience psychiatric symptoms like depression and anxiety, or they feel dizzy and have frequent headaches. These symptoms happen because the neurological system is lacking the fuel it needs to function properly. If glucose is the "fuel" that your nervous system needs to run on and the fuel gauge begins flashing "low," (there's that check engine light again) problems are going to surface. Essentially, your body's fuel source becomes so low that your neurons can't fire properly and begin losing function. Your car runs out of gas.

On the flip side, when there's an excess of glucose in the body, it's like taking sandpaper to the outside of an electrical cord. Inside the plastic sheath of the cord, there's a metal wire, which conducts electricity, just like our nervous system. If you take sandpaper to that coating and rub through the outer sheath, you can't put the protective sheath back on, leaving the bare wire exposed.

Too much glucose in the body has the same effect on the myelin sheath surrounding your nerve fibers. Myelin is an insulating layer that forms around nerves, including those in the brain and spinal cord. It is made up of protein and fatty substances, and it allows electrical impulses to transmit quickly and efficiently along the nerve cells. If that myelin coating is worn through, it can't be replaced as long as your glucose level is high. Once the nerve is exposed, the body's electrical system starts to malfunction because it lacks the protection it needs.

An excess of glucose can also cause balance problems, stability problems, coordination issues, and trouble with focus, attention, and concentration. Extreme cases of hyperglycemia can also cause kidney malfunction, blindness, or require the amputation of limbs. When there is too much glucose present in the bloodstream, things like insulin resistance start to appear, which is the precursor to diabetes. Interestingly enough, "Type 3" diabetes, a proposed term to describe the interlinked association between Type 1 and Type 2 diabetes and Alzheimer's disease, is also known as dementia and occurs when neurons in the brain become unable to respond to insulin, which is essential for basic tasks, including memory and learning.

Whether you are hypoglycemic (too little glucose) or hyperglycemic (too much glucose), the reality is that neither condition is ideal. Balanced, stable blood sugar levels are the goal, and when you get your glucose leveled out, everything begins to improve. You may even begin sleeping better because REM cycles are affected by both hyper and hypoglycemia. Your overall body function may improve, especially your liver, kidney, bladder and digestive health. How and why? Your organ system has to communicate with your brain and your brain has to communicate with your organs and it does this through the Vagus Nerve. With balanced blood sugar, you'll enjoy more energy and less mental and physical fatigue.

YOUR FIRST STEPS

When I see patients, I'm looking for an optimal fasting glucose level on their blood panel of anywhere from 85-99 and A1C below 5.3. This is different from the "medical normal" range which is 70-110. When I see a patient over 99, I consider them pre-diabetic because at this level, insulin resistance is already starting to destroy their nerve function, brain function, blood vessel function and organ function. When a person hits 126, they've officially entered into a disease process known as diabetes.

Anything below 85 is hypoglycemia meaning there's too little glucose in your blood for the neurological system to run at its peak level. If hypoglycemia gets to an advanced stage, it can actually cause you to pass out because there's such a severe lack of fuel that your neurons can't fire.

Your first step to balancing your blood sugar and stabilizing your glucose levels is to understand how and why you got to where you are today. Here's where I'm going to give you some tough love. Unless you are a Type 1 diabetic (which is an autoimmune disorder), this Type 2 diabetes is a self-inflicted condition. You did this to yourself. Ouch, I know that's hard to hear. The good news is that you can also undo it! This is where personal responsibility really comes into play.

To immediately begin stabilizing your glucose levels, I encourage you to start moving. Exercise burns off glucose, stimulates your nervous system, and increases your body's oxygen levels. Win, win, and win! Start with simple forms of movement like walking or bicycling, and then work up to more strenuous activities like swimming, workout classes, or weight lifting. Regardless of where you're at in your health journey, find a form of exercise that you enjoy and start doing it. Try to move your body every day. Again, motion is life! If you rest, you rust.

The second key to stabilizing your blood sugar is found in the kitchen. It's all about what you put in your mouth. What you put in your mouth is just as important as the way you move your body. Start tracking your food using a phone app like MyFitnessPal to find out how many grams of carbs and sugar you're consuming each day. You don't have to track your food forever, but committing to it for 60-90 days is one of the best tools to teach you how to eat properly. Most people are shocked when they see their initial numbers. Get rid of the bread, cake, and cookies. Eat less carbs and consume more healthy proteins and fats (baked chicken, fish, bison). Portion sizes are also crucial. Measure out your meals carefully and skip on seconds.

Glucose is essential for solving chronic health problems because it's the fuel that our neurological system needs to do its job. However, having too much or too little glucose can cause serious health issues and even create serious disease processes like diabetes. Doing these simple things can help you conquer your goal of achieving long-term health through stable glucose levels. Now that we've talked about glucose, let's move on to the next key to solving chronic health problems - stimulation.

CHAPTER 7

KEY 3 – STIMULATION

THE ROLE OF STIMULATION

The definition of neurostimulation is "the activation of a nerve through an external source." Touch, for example, is a kind of stimulation as well as walking, cycling or swimming. Seeing something new is a form of stimulation. Hearing your friend speak is a form of stimulation. Picking up a 5lb weight and doing a bicep curl is a type of stimulation. When it comes to the neurological system, neural pathways need stimulation in order to be healthy. These pathways are designed to send information and signals (both electrically and chemically) from the body to the brain and the brain to the body, and don't forget your organ system is part of your body. Think of the neurological system like a muscle. If it's stimulated, it grows and gets stronger. If it's not stimulated, it begins to atrophy just like a muscle that isn't used enough.

It's crucial to understand the role that stimulation plays in solving chronic health problems because this is an area of health that's so often overlooked. Stimulation is required to stabilize neurological function. When a system is under-stimulated, it begins to atrophy and so does the area of the brain that controls that body part. To solve this problem, I use targeted, specific types of stimulation to "fire" those pathways. This activation creates more neuro-plasticity and increases the function of that area of the neurological systems. Neuro-plasticity (also known as "brain plasticity") is the ability of the brain and nervous system to modify its connections or rewire itself. Stimulating certain areas of the nervous system in specific ways makes the brain fire better which can solve problems in the body.

Different parts of the body are connected to different parts of the brain. For instance, if you are having problems with smell, taste, memory, or vision, all of those senses fire through your temporal lobe which means that part of your brain needs a certain kind of stimulation to get it working again. The reason we have to understand stimulation is because we need to find out what part of the brain is malfunctioning and figure out which systems we need to stimulate to bring that part of the brain back online.

For example, if a patient breaks their arm, their arm is going to atrophy within two weeks. They can eat broccoli and cauliflower and asparagus every day, five times per day, but if they don't stimulate the arm muscles, they're going to get smaller. The only way to make this muscle grow is to stimulate it. Specifically, a person with a broken arm, once the arm is out of the cast, needs the stimulation of bicep curls and tricep extensions to bring it and the part of their brain that controls their arm back to full working capacity. Doing calf raises, even though it's a form of stimulation, wouldn't help heal their arm because it's the wrong kind of stimulation. This method is known as "receptor-based activation," and it uses movement and stimulation to activate the brain.

Certain parts of the brain perform certain functions and control specific parts of the body. When we experience problems in our body, it's often because certain parts of the brain are not functioning as they should. Stimulating different parts of the brain in specific ways makes it "fire" or signal better which in turn solves problems in the body, and some of the stories that have come from treating patients through receptor-based activation have been nothing short of amazing.

A few years ago, a man came into the clinic and was having a major shoulder problem. In fact, his shoulder movement was so poor that he could barely get his arms to the level of his shoulders. He'd been to five different doctors and undergone many different forms of treatment, yet nothing had helped him move his arms normally. After I talked with him and did a neurological examination, it became clear that he needed receptor-based activation in his flexion / extension muscle groups. We worked together for several minutes and immediately afterwards, he was able to move his arms all the way over his head without any assistance. Why did this treatment work so fast? Because stimulating the correct area of the brain helped it become balanced, and it functioned more optimally because of it. Correct neurological stimulation is an amazing modality.

RESULTS OF STIMULATION

What actually happens when the body has a deficiency of stimulation? To understand the inner workings of the human brain, we first need to wrap our minds around the massive amount of energy that it requires to operate. The brain weighs about three pounds, and it is very metabolically demanding, consuming 25-30% of our overall oxygen and glucose intake. Consider that for a moment. Almost one third of the oxygen and glucose brought into our bodies is used by the brain alone. It is by far the most energy demanding organ, and because of that, the brain requires a constant supply of oxygen and glucose.

If the brain has the right amounts of oxygen and glucose, the final key that it needs to maintain optimal health is - you guessed it - proper neurological stimulation. It's the final piece of the Big Three (oxygen, glucose, stimulation) for maintaining a healthy, vibrant neurological system. If there's a lack of stimulation, the neurons will begin to break down and no longer produce the electrical and chemical activation to maintain neuronal health, which in turn causes the neurological pathways to atrophy. The atrophy of the pathways also causes atrophy in the brain. If you don't use it you lose it. In order for the neurological system to be healthy, it must be stimulated. If you want your arms to be strong, you have to do push-ups. If you don't, you'll have skinny, weak arms. If you don't stimulate your brain and neurological pathways, they break down as well, and the first signs of loss of brain health is brain fog, and the loss of focus, attention and concentration.

If the idea of your brain atrophying and your neurological pathways malfunctioning doesn't sound pleasant, I have good news for you. There may be a solution to your problem! You can increase the level of neurological stimulation and improve your health in a multitude of ways. When you increase stimulation in your daily life, you may experience an increased memory capacity, better vision, a clearer memory, a better sense of taste and smell, and more appreciation for touch. With all of these exciting benefits to gain, let's dig into strategies for self-testing and improving stimulation in your daily life.

YOUR FIRST STEPS -
EVALUATION AND STIMULATION

There are several simple ways to test the health of your neurological pathways. The first indicator of a healthy brain is your ability to learn new information, to stay focused, and to concentrate on the topic at hand. When is the last time you learned something for the first time? The only long-term way to maintain the health of your brain is to stimulate it by trying new things, tasting new foods, smelling new smells, seeing new sights, and going to new places. Pay attention to how mentally "rigid" you are towards new ideas or plans. People who are inflexible and have a "my way or the highway" mentality often have very unhealthy brains.

When I examine the health of a patient's brain, there are four main areas of the brain that I consider: the temporal lobe, the parietal lobe, the frontal lobe, and the prefrontal lobe (or prefrontal cortex). The temporal lobe controls taste, smell, memory, and vision. The parietal lobe is in charge of body sensation and vision. The frontal lobe controls voluntary movement, and the prefrontal cortex handles focus, attention, concentration, memory, impulse control, and motivation. The deficiency of stimulation also determines which part of the brain is malfunctioning, and this is all determined through neurological testing. I have many tests that I do at my clinic, but there are also easy, at-home testing strategies for each lobe of the brain.

Temporal lobe self-test: Ask yourself these questions: "Can I taste and smell things as I did before? Have my senses increased, decreased or stayed the same? (If they've decreased, that indicates a lack of stimulation in the temporal lobe). How's my memory? Am I as "sharp" as ever or has my memory declined?"

Parietal lobe self-test: One simple test is called the Digit Span Test. Here's how you perform it. You need a partner. Close your eyes and have your partner touch two of your toes on one foot. Can you identify how many toes are between the toes your partner is touching? Now repeat on the other foot as well as your fingers on both hands. If this neurological system is damaged, you will not be able to identify what your partner is doing.

Frontal lobe self-test: Do I move as well now as I did in the past or has my movement slowed? How is my memory compared to years past? Am I becoming more irritated over trivial things? Am I becoming more inflexible? The biggest problem with frontal lobe issues is that you don't see the change but everyone around you does. It's strange but with frontal lobe demise, we can't see it in ourselves but everyone else can see our deficiencies.

Prefrontal cortex self-test: A healthy prefrontal cortex is essential for planning, and execution of complex issues such as behavior, speech, and logical reasoning, as well as impulse control, motivation, understanding the consequences of your actions, and short term memory. If you've noticed you're not following through with what you've started, planning poorly, having short term memory as well as lacking impulse control, then your prefrontal cortex may need some rehab.

CEREBELLUM:

Stability test (do this with caution): Put your feet together (side-by-side), close your eyes, and hold that position for 15 seconds. Next, put your right foot in front of the left, close your eyes and hold for 15 seconds. Lastly, put your left foot in front of your right foot, close your eyes, and hold for 15 seconds.

Flex test (do this with caution): Stand on one leg with the other leg lifted and flexed at 90 degrees, then hold that position for 15 seconds. Repeat on the other side.

These cerebellar tests are very important for stability and balance. Count out loud and see how long you can maintain your balance and stability. A healthy cerebellum will allow for the full fifteen seconds for each test.

These simple at-home tests can give you an idea of how your neurological pathways are currently firing, and if you performed the tests and didn't like the results, don't fear. Here are some exercises you can do to stimulate those pathways and "fire" your brain back up.

Non-linear complex movements: You can actually do these exercises while you're sitting down at the table or relaxing on your couch. Start by sitting down or standing up, then do a figure eight in the air with your arm or "write" the name of your city and state in the air, write your ABCs, your name, etc. Try writing your name in the air with your hand and leg at the same time. This fires your cerebellum, frontal lobe and the parietal lobe at that same time. Pair this with deep breathing and you're really stimulating your brain and giving it plenty of oxygen to increase the level of stimulation your neurological system can take.

Deep breathing exercises: As stated before deep breathing or forced breathing stimulates frontal lobe function. Start slowly and build up and remember the 1:2 ratio. Breathe in four seconds and out eight seconds. Once you can perform 4:8 move up to 6:12, six seconds in and twelve seconds out. Next step is 8:16, eight seconds in and sixteen seconds out. It won't be easy getting to 8:16 but remember, things worth having are hardly ever easy.

CHAPTER 8

KEY 4 – AUTOIMMUNE DISORDERS

THE ROLE OF AUTOIMMUNE (AI) DISORDERS

Before we dig into autoimmune disorders and their profound impact on your health, let's first look at the driver of autoimmunity which is your immune system. So what is an immune system, exactly, and why is it important to your body? Your immune system is basically your built-in SEAL Team 6. It's your body's special defense mechanism against all of the antigens of the world. An antigen is any substance that sparks your immune system to produce antibodies such as chemicals, bacteria, cancer cells, viruses, or pollen. Your immune system recognizes that these antigens are not meant to be inside of you and then activates to fight off and kill the offender. When you develop an autoimmune condition, your immune system begins attacking your own tissues because it thinks your tissue is the antigen. Essentially, an autoimmune condition is "friendly fire" within your body.

Autoimmune (AI) conditions can be devastating to patients suffering with chronic health problems because AI can not only exacerbate existing chronic problems, but AI by itself is the health problem. The autoimmune condition acts like the Tasmanian devil inside your body, wreaking havoc and causing damage. Once an autoimmune condition begins destroying things, it can cause a whole host of other seemingly unrelated issues.

One of the biggest drivers of autoimmune conditions that I see in my clinic is a sensitivity to gluten. Gluten is a protein found in wheat and is in manufactured cereal, grains, pasta, bread and flour, just to name a few products. It is the substance that makes bread dough elastic and stretchy, and it is devastating to the human brain. Gluten is one of the most destructive proteins found on the planet today, and no, it's not the same wheat that our ancestors consumed centuries ago. It's a commercialized, hybridized version that our body can no longer recognize or break down. As a result, undigested gluten proteins work their way into the bloodstream and spark an immune response. Since gluten's amino acid profile closely resembles the amino acid profile of the human thyroid gland and cerebellum tissue, this immune response quickly turns into an autoimmune response that attacks those parts of your body.

Every single human needs to test their tolerance for gluten, and the test I recommend is panel A2 from www.Enterolab. com. You can order this test directly from the company. Another test is Cyrex Array 3, but a doctor has to order this test. This is a genetic test which identifies whether or not you carry the gluten sensitivity gene and if it has been turned on. It also tells you whether or not you have the Celiac gene. I can't stress enough how important it is for everyone to become educated on gluten intolerance and their body's reaction to wheat and other cereal grains.

RESULTS FROM AUTOIMMUNE DISORDERS

When your body is battling an autoimmune disorder, it could appear as a multitude of other, seemingly unrelated chronic health problems. Ataxia, which is an unstable posture or irregular gait, is commonly linked to autoimmune disease. Thyroid problems like Hashimoto's Disease can be rooted in autoimmune conditions. Recent research has suggested approximately 90% of people who have thyroid issues also have an autoimmune disorder. Fibromyalgia is a chronic disorder characterized by widespread musculoskeletal pain, fatigue, and tenderness in localized areas and is often rooted in autoimmune problems. Cerebellum issues like blurred vision, balance problems, and uncoordinated movements with your hands and feet are all signals that you may be dealing with an autoimmune condition.

Other signs of autoimmune disease are general cognitive decline like a lack of focus, attention and concentration. Dementia, forgetting things like names, numbers, and dates, is a concerning signal of an autoimmune condition. Psychological disorders like panic, anxiety, depression, and irrational fear are often rooted in autoimmune causes as well. Migraine headaches, multiple sclerosis, ALS (often called Lou Gehrig's disease), stiffness in movements, tremors, and restless leg syndrome are all chronic conditions that are closely linked to autoimmune roots with the majority of these reactions being triggered by the gluten found in modern wheat.

Many people mistakenly think that only people diagnosed with Celiac disease are intolerant to gluten, however the truth is that only about 30% of people who have Celiac disease have gut-related issues. The other 70% have a myriad of other problems.

Celiac disease destroys the microvilli, the tiny hair-like projections within the small intestine that increase nutrient absorption. These projections increase the surface area of the small intestine allowing more area for nutrients to be absorbed. Celiac destroys these microvilli to the point that they can't absorb nutrients. When they are damaged, it kicks off a host of other disease processes that can turn into full-blown autoimmune conditions.

YOUR FIRST STEP

When the gut becomes inflamed and damaged, harmful proteins like gluten cross the blood-brain barrier and "dock" in the part of your brain where your opioid receptors live. This means people who regularly eat breads, cakes, cookies, brownies, and other foods containing wheat flour are truly addicted to these foods. When they eat them, their brain reacts very similarly to someone consuming opioids. What's your reaction as you've read my encouragement to ditch wheat and gluten? Did you say, "No way! I can't live without my (fill in the blank)." If those thoughts crossed your mind, there's a good chance you're addicted to gluten.

I can't encourage you strongly enough - get gluten out of your life. The side effects are absolutely devastating. If you want to learn more about the bad effects of gluten, I highly recommend the book *Grain Brain* by David Perlmutter, MD. It goes into much more detail on the effects that modern gluten has on the human brain.

If you suspect that you have a lurking autoimmune condition, don't lose hope. It may be possible to slow down the damage, and in some cases even reverse it IF caught early enough. Here comes "tough love part two." The most important point for you to remember is this: improving the lives of patients suffering with chronic health problems begins with my patients taking personal responsibility. Most autoimmune conditions are triggered by lifestyle choices which means that they can also be improved upon through major lifestyle changes. These kinds of changes can be challenging to make, but what is your health worth to you? That's the question you need to answer when you look in the mirror, "Am I worth it?" Only you can answer that question.

The first step to identifying an autoimmune condition is to order the www.EnteroLab.com panel A2 test. If I was a betting kind of guy, I would wager that you do have the gluten sensitivity gene. If you have a gluten sensitivity problem, it's crucial that you avoid gluten at all costs and get on an autoimmune paleo diet. You also need to start the Brain-Body-Gut 10-week detox program.

Will you make mistakes? Absolutely! Anyone taking on a major lifestyle change will slip up and fall off "the bandwagon" as we say, but don't let those mistakes keep you from getting back on the program. Keep heading in the right direction and you will begin to see improvement.

A great first step in the right direction is to deep clean your home of all products containing gluten. This includes cooking devices like toasters that have touched your bread, English muffins, etc. Throw away all wheat flours, breads, cookies, baking mixes, and more. With a wheat and gluten sensitivity, you're either all in or you're out. You can't be 95% in, you have to be 100% committed because once you consume gluten, it takes months for it to completely leave your system.

Take heart. There is hope. You can get rid of all the negative side effects of gluten while still enjoying your life. However, it takes time and commitment for these changes to become part of your new lifestyle. If you're willing to put in the work, I can almost guarantee you'll see a significant improvement in your health. Now that we've covered autoimmune disorders, let's move to the next key to solving chronic health problems.

CHAPTER 9

KEY 5 – INFLAMMATION

THE ROLE OF INFLAMMATION

Inflammation - this is a term we hear often, but do we really know what it is, why it happens, and why we often have too much of it? Let's start by discussing what inflammation is supposed to do. In its proper context, inflammation is actually a good thing because it acts as a signaling agent to tell the body to start repairing, restoring, and regenerating itself. This regeneration is kicked off by the formation of new blood vessels. Nothing can heal until new blood vessels are created (called angiogenesis), and in this regard, inflammation is a positive thing.

Inflammation comes to the rescue when you experience an acute injury like a twisted ankle, a dislocated shoulder, or a badly banged shin. In that context, inflammation is a localized physical condition that causes the body to become swollen, red, and hot to the touch. This is when inflammation signals to the rest of the body to begin the healing process. The trouble begins when inflammation gets out of hand and out of homeostasis.

Homeostasis is the body's ability to maintain a relatively stable internal state that persists despite changes in the world outside. When there isn't homeostasis, disease processes can begin to develop. As with many parts of our health, inflammation causes problems when it goes rogue and there is too much of it.

Inflammation becomes a major issue when it's continually present in the body. This can happen for a variety of reasons. In this scenario, inflammation in the body is like fire inside of a house. It's totally destructive and stands in the way of optimizing chronic issues. Some of the most common signs of chronic inflammation are actually more psychological than physical. Brain fog, depression, anxiety, irritability, and fatigue are all signs of chronic inflammation of the brain. When chronic inflammation exists in the brain, that dreaded brain fog is almost always the first symptom to appear. Sometimes I compare it to feeling like the "walking dead" or like you're living in zombie land. You have a hard time focusing, concentrating, and staying hooked on one task for an extended period of time.

Inflammation plays a distinct and important role in healing chronic disease because it's something we must eliminate before we can begin untangling the web of dysfunction and healing the root issue. If a house was on fire, would you start rebuilding it before the fire was completely put out? No, that would be ridiculous. In the same way, we have to eradicate the chronic inflammation before we can begin rebuilding the body. If there's chronic inflammation present, it's going to accelerate the degeneration in your brain, joints, nervous system, and circulatory system much more quickly. If you're dealing with any kind of inflammation anywhere, you have to zap it before you can start to heal.

Bloodwork is the most accurate way to measure the level of inflammation present in the body. The A1C markers on a blood panel can be used to measure inflammation. The CRP (c-reactive protein) and the homocysteine markers also indicate inflammation levels. Everyone has some level of inflammation present in their system at all times, but these tests are used to see if it is out of control or not. This information is used to make a plan for reducing the level of chronic inflammation in your system.

RESULTS OF INFLAMMATION

So what causes this kind of chronic inflammation? The factors can be both psychological and physical. Psychological things like being overworked, excessively difficult workouts, unhealthy relationships, a stressful job, and not having enough "me time" can all contribute to chronic inflammation of the brain.

Physical causes of chronic inflammation can be obvious things like slipping and falling, a car wreck (even if it was several years ago), whiplash, repetitive injuries or motions, falling out of a tree, falling off a ladder, and more. Chronic inflammation from these kinds of traumatic injuries can stay with you many years, even after the more obvious symptoms disappear.

A glucose imbalance (see Chapter 6), anemia, leaky gut syndrome, leaky brain syndrome, and food sensitivities can cause out-of-control inflammation in the body. When these things occur, the body releases cortisol to combat the stress of the inflammatory process. Cortisol is a stress-related hormone that is meant to help control blood sugar levels, regulate metabolism, help reduce inflammation, and assist with memory formulation. However, when the body signals cortisol to be released over and over again, the negative effects begin to spiral out of control. If there's too much cortisol in your system, it can affect the quality of your sleep. It also directly attacks the hippocampus, the region of the brain that is associated primarily with memory.

Decreasing the level of inflammation in your system will positively affect your health in many, many ways. First of all, it will save your brain. That sounds extreme, but it's true. The brain is very sensitive to inflammation, and by decreasing the level of inflammation in the brain, you're going to avoid many memory, focus and concentration, and anxiety driven problems. When you put out the "fire in the house," your focus, attention, and brain fog should significantly decrease. You should have an increased ability to think more clearly and experience a clarity of mind and senses that you haven't noticed for quite a while. As you work to decrease the inflammation in your body, your pain syndromes should start to decrease. Your joint pain may slow down or be completely eliminated, and you may even notice your balance improving.

If your inflammation levels are out of control, the first thing to do is look at is your diet. You can take all the anti-inflammatory products in the world, but you can't out-supplement a poor diet. You can't out-medicate it either. Making the necessary dietary changes (most commonly, eliminating gluten, sugar, and casein, the protein found in milk) is a major first step to reducing inflammation and healing chronic disease.

YOUR FIRST STEPS

So what can you do, starting today, to begin decreasing the inflammation level in your body? What a great question! The exciting thing is that there is a lot you can do to help put out the fire and set the stage for true healing. First let's talk about psychological and physiological things you can do to reduce one of the biggest drivers of inflammation, which is stress.

If you notice stress playing a major inflammatory role in your life, start incorporating important mental health practices like regular deep tissue massage and "unplugging" from technology on a regular basis. No one is going to care more about your brain and bodily health than you, and you need to make these things a major priority in your life. All of these things are an investment in your long-term health. Make a commitment to disconnect from technology for one day per week. Schedule a ninety minute massage once per month. Listen to soothing music. Go to a happy, funny movie and laugh for a whole hour straight. Listen to soothing nature sounds. Eliminate the bad and unnecessarily stressful relationships from your life. If you're in a bad relationship, discontinue it or take the hard but necessary steps to improve it. All of these small changes add up to a major effect. It's like a snowball that's rolling down a hill. At first, the changes seem minor, but as you pick up speed, the momentum becomes undeniable.

As far as physical changes that can help decrease inflammation, there are a lot of them. First of all, stop eating gluten, casein, and sugar. These substances do nothing but cause inflammation and wreak havoc on your gut-brain health. Stop eating processed foods that are filled with inflammatory oils and Trans Fats. Examples of trans fats include, but are not limited to, store bought cakes, cookies and pies, shortening, microwave popcorn, frozen pizza, fried foods, doughnuts, non-dairy creamer, and margarine. No wonder you're having headaches, brain fog and your feet are tingling and numb. In addition to dietary changes, you can incorporate other physical things like using an inversion table or adding nutritional supplements into your daily routine.

I think everyone should be taking an omega-3 fish oil supplement, and lots of it. The bare minimum daily required amount is 500mg but you can take up to 5000mg with zero negative side effects. Take the best kind you can afford. If you've had a bad experience with Omega-3 supplements in the past, it may be because you took a poor quality supplement. Up your intake of foods high in antioxidants, aka super foods. This includes things like purple, red or blue grapes (make sure they have seeds in them and eat the seeds as well), blueberries, raspberries, raw almonds, walnuts, pecans, kale, spinach (see, Popeye was right), broccoli, sweet potatoes, green or black tea, beans, and fish. These substances help rid the body of free radicals caused by inflammation. Drink real home-brewed green tea. Choose a high-quality whole leaf (or loose leaf) green tea that is organic and minimally processed.

When you begin to incorporate these lifestyle changes into your daily routine, you will be amazed at the way your body and brain feel. Eliminating inflammation in your body is a fantastic step toward healing chronic health problems and regaining your health and vibrancy. Now that we've talked about inflammation, let's move onto the next key - environmental toxins.

CHAPTER 10

KEY 6 – NEUROTOXINS

THE ROLE OF NEUROTOXINS

A neurotoxin is something you ingest into your body that has a direct link to brain and neurological destruction. The word "neurotoxin" may spark images of strange green substances bubbling in chemistry class, but the reality is that neurotoxins are hiding in some of the most ingested substances on earth. In fact, you probably have many of these substances in your kitchen right now, and understanding the role these toxins play in either starting or continuing chronic health problems is crucial. As your body digests and breaks down a neurotoxic substance, it may either trigger an autoimmune attack or kick off some kind of destructive brain and/or body disease process.

Here's a list of the most common neurotoxins that the majority of Americans consume every day:

- Wheat, particularly the gluten (the protein found in wheat), is the most destructive protein you can ever put in your body therefore it is classified as a neurotoxin. Again, I recommend the book *Grain Brain* by David Perlmutter, MD.

- Common table sugar is also a neurotoxin. As your body breaks it down, your blood sugar becomes spiked, which triggers a release of insulin which in turn produces a destructive inflammatory response.

- High fructose corn syrup is highly inflammatory. Most commonly used as a sweetener in sodas and other sweet drinks, high fructose corn syrup triggers a similar inflammatory response as table sugar. Because of this, I highly suggest you stop drinking sodas immediately.

- Artificial sweeteners are very toxic to the brain. Though they seem innocent because they don't contain sugar, they harm the brain in a different way. They contain a substance that causes our bodies' glutamate, an excitatory neurotransmitter, to over react to the product. It's similar to slamming the gas pedal of your car to the floor while it's in park and over-revving the engine to the point of blowing it up. These artificial sweeteners do the same thing to your glutamate neurotransmitters and essentially blow their doors off. To avoid artificial sweeteners, stop drinking diet soda as well as other diet beverages.

- Monosodium Glutamate (MSG) is another substance that has a similar effect on your sensory neurotransmitters as the artificial sweeteners. This substance over-excites those receptors to the point of malfunction and degeneration which then leads to negative psychological side effects like brain fog, depression, and anxiety. To avoid MSG, steer clear of processed foods like flavored tortilla chips, ranch dressing mixes, some soy sauces and prepackaged Asian foods, and other highly processed items.

- Trans fats are hydrogenated oils that are highly inflammatory to the body. Anything that is inflammatory over a long period of time is going to destroy your brain function so avoiding anything that contains trans fats is crucial.

- Drinking bottled water from the commonly sold plastic disposable bottles has proven to be a source of neurotoxic material. Avoiding the consumption of and exposure to these plastic products greatly reduces the toxic load on your body's detoxification systems.

- There are a few more common neurotoxic culprits like heavy metals - lead, mercury, and formaldehyde, and these toxic substances are found in some unsuspecting places. Recent medical studies have shown that lead poisoning may be generational. The results showed that if a parent got lead poisoning, it took roughly 4 generations to get it out of their offspring's system. Mercury (aka thermasol) is found in vaccines, as well as aluminum, which is in most underarm deodorants.

RESULTS FROM NEUROTOXINS

Understanding the realities and effects of neurotoxins plays an important role in helping people optimize their chronic issues. Since these neurotoxins damage the brain, the body's most important healing organ, it only stands to reason that removing substances which hurt the brain will accelerate healing. When there's a large amount of neurotoxins present in your body, it accelerates the degeneration of your joints, causes focus and concentration issues, can increase fear and anxiety, activate autoimmune disorders and destroy body tissue. Many chronic diseases, movement disorders, fibromyalgia, burning and numbness, tingling and coordination problems can be linked to an overload of neurotoxins.

These negative effects are often overlooked because most people, even traditional doctors, don't understand the link between inflammation of the brain and one's ability to improve their chronic condition. A brain and body detox as well as an elimination diet are very useful tools for changing your body's chemistry and your lifestyle so you can kick these nasty toxins to the curb.

Decreasing your consumption of neurotoxins will also yield some very nice lifestyle benefits like better sleep (the more cortisol you have, the less melatonin you release therefore making it harder to fall asleep and stay asleep), decreased pain and discomfort, better bowel movements, improved sexual function, better concentration and focus, and greater stability and balance.

YOUR FIRST STEPS

Your first step is to remember that you have the power to stop eating, drinking, and surrounding yourself with foods and substances that are neurotoxic to your brain. Stop eating the processed foods and quit drinking sodas, both traditional and diet.

Stop buying plastic water bottles and instead invest in a glass water bottle that you refill at home with reverse osmosis water. If you have coffee, make sure you drink only organic coffee. Flavor your water with lemon or lime juice instead of ingesting traditional soda drinks or artificial sweeteners. There are many, many ways to enjoy the things you love like a great cup of coffee or a refreshing beverage without sacrificing your health.

The bottom line is to eliminate the neurotoxins listed above. Are there other toxins out there besides the ones I talked about in this book? Absolutely. There are herbicides, pesticides, environmental toxins, and more, but your exposure to those are mostly out of your control. Instead of focusing on what we can't control, let's focus on what we can control. You get to control everything you put in your mouth and on your body. Those daily choices are either healing you or slowly killing you, and you get to decide which direction you choose.

CHAPTER 11

KEY 7 – THE BRAIN-GUT CONNECTION

THE ROLE OF GUT HEALTH

What is your "gut?" What does it have to do with healing chronic disease and untangling the web of dysfunction? Why does the condition of your gut matter so much for your overall health picture? How is gut health connected to the well-being of your brain? We're going to answer all of these important questions and more in this chapter.

For starters, your "gut" is not referring to the roundness we get around our midsection when we eat too many Christmas cookies. Instead, the term "gut health" refers to the physical state and physiologic function of the many parts of the gastrointestinal tract, also called the Enteric Nervous System. At one time, our digestive system was considered a relatively "simple" body system, but as our understanding of the gut and its many functions has grown, it's proven to be anything but simple. The gut not only consists of many different organs which work together to withdraw nutrition from our food, it also is home to trillions of microorganisms which live in our intestines. These microorganisms are a mixture of beneficial and non-beneficial bacteria, and in a healthy, optimally functioning gut, the "good bugs" far outnumber the "bad bugs." What's even more amazing is that these microorganisms are an essential part of your immune system, and over 70% of your immune system is found in your gut. The health and wellness of these microorganisms greatly depends on the foods we eat, the stress we endure, the medications we take, and the environment we live in.

In recent years, more attention has been paid to the importance of gut health and the way an unhealthy gut contributes to the web of dysfunction. The gut is so crucial to our overall wellness for more reasons than digesting food and extracting nutrients. Your gut (Enteric Nervous System) is connected to your brain via the Vagus Nerve, and in fact, they're so connected that we should almost view them as one system. If one is damaged, dysfunction in the other is sure to follow.

The link between the gut and the brain is known as the "gut/brain axis." The two are so interconnected that they're basically one, ultra complex system. The human gut (Enteric Nervous System) is lined with more than 500 million nerve cells so it's practically a brain unto itself. To give you an example, the human spinal cord has approximately 100 million nerve cells. Because the Gut/Brain axis is so interconnected, in order to heal one, you have to also heal the other. The neuro-metabolic web of dysfunction really starts to untangle when you solve the problems with your Gut/Brain Axis.

There are two main ways that the brain and the gut communicate with one another, and either of these modes of communication can be disrupted by trauma or inflammation. The first way the brain and gut communicate is through the Vagus nerve, a large "super highway" kind of nerve that extends from the brain stem to part of the colon. It also happens to be the longest cranial nerve in the body.

The second way the gut and the brain communicate is through the Central Autonomic Network which is also known as the

"C.A.N." This complex network can be compromised by trauma as well as physiological or psychological issues. Any kind of damage to either the function of the Vagus nerve or the C.A.N. may spark leaky gut syndrome in your body. In fact, research suggests that within 6-12 hours after trauma happens to the brain (concussion, whiplash injury), you will have a leaky gut.

Your digestive system plays a key role in protecting your body from harmful substances. The walls of the intestines act as barriers, kind of like screen doors in our home, controlling what enters the bloodstream to be transported to your organs. If that screen is compromised, the barrier is breached and bugs get into the house. We have these kinds of protective barriers in our brain and gut and when they're damaged, trouble occurs. The inflammatory cascade starts here.

Small gaps in the intestinal wall called "tight junctions" allow water and nutrients to pass through, while blocking the passage of harmful substances. When these tight junctions are damaged to the point that they open up and no longer prevent harmful substances from passing into the bloodstream, it is known as "leaky gut syndrome." Leaky gut can be summarized in two words – intestinal permeability. When the gut is "leaky" and bacteria and other antigens enter the bloodstream, it can cause widespread inflammation and potentially trigger a reaction from the immune system. Those harmful substances are supposed to simply pass through the digestive tract, and when they breach that barrier and get into your bloodstream, they wreak all kinds of havoc.

Gluten sensitivity as well as an overload of neurotoxins can also cause damage and result in a leaky gut. The reason that gut health is so crucial is because if your gut isn't healthy and doing its job, it affects every other system in the body. To solve the riddle of chronic health issues and begin to untangle the neuro-metabolic web of dysfunction, we have to address brain function and gut function. That's why gut health is one of my seven keys to healing chronic health issues.

Gut health plays a distinct role in fostering true health and healing chronic disease because of the key role it plays in your immune system. As I mentioned earlier, about 70% of your immune system is found in your gut. To foster true health, you also need homeostasis between your sympathetic and parasympathetic nervous systems. Your Vagus nerve, the nerve that runs from the brainstem all the way to the colon, is what controls all of these functions.

To measure your gut health, there are several good blood work tests that show whether your gut is functioning correctly or not. The www.EnteroLab.com panel A2 test indicates if the gut is functioning properly. If you have an immune response to milk, wheat, soy or eggs, you likely have a leaky gut. If you have a leaky gut, you have a leaky brain.

RESULTS FROM GUT HEALTH

When you have poor gut health, there are a whole host of problems that could be showing up in your life. Some of the physical maladies you may be experiencing include GERD (gastroesophageal reflux disease), Crohn's disease, irritable bowel syndrome, SIBO (small intestinal bacterial overgrowth), and gastric reflux. These common disease processes all find their roots in having a leaky gut.

Many psychological issues like brain fog, lack of focus and attention, depression, anxiety, and overwhelming fear can develop as a result of leaky gut because when the gut is not healthy, neither is the brain. As I said before, you cannot have a healthy brain unless you have a healthy gut. If you have damage to the brain or you're feeding your gut bad stuff, those barriers are compromised and it kicks off a wave of inflammation and autoimmune disorders.

YOUR FIRST STEPS

So what can you do, starting today, to increase your gut health?

1. Eliminate the seven most common neurotoxins (see chapter 10). If you damage your brain, you damage your gut and vice versa.

2. Complete the Brain-Body-Gut 10-week detox program. Detoxifying your body and supporting your gut and brain health will kick start your path to healing and help you begin to untangle the web of dysfunction.

3. Do the nerve stimulation exercises below 3-4 times per week. Since the Vagus nerve is the main super highway which allows the gut and brain to communicate, stimulating the Vagus nerve regularly is a fantastic way to promote optimal gut health.

I also suggest some extremely high quality nutritional supplements. The supplements listed below are NOT FDA approved to treat and disease or cure any aliment, and is NOT to take the place of any medication your doctor may have prescribed.

i. *Apex Energetics – ClearVite-PSF (K-84) Part 1 of 3 of our Brain-Body-Gut 10-week detox program. Helps support liver detoxification reactions, the biliary system, and sugar metabolism.*

ii. *Apex Energetics – RepairVite (K-60) Part 2 of 3 of our Brain-Body-Gut 10-week detox program. Intended to support the intestinal tract and intestinal lining.*

iii. *Apex Energetics – Strengtia Probiotics (K-61) Part 3 of 3 of our Brain-Body-Gut 10-week detox program. Designed to fortify the intestinal microbial environment with targeted probiotics.*

iv. *Apex Energetics – Omega-CO3 (K-7) intended to support the brain and the immune system.*

v. *Apex Energetics – Protoglysen (K-28) and Glysen (K-1) Both are designed to support sugar metabolism and help buffer glycemic response.*

vi. *Apex Energetics - NeurO2 (K-45) uniquely designed and mechanistically balanced to support the cerebral microvascular for healthy blood flow to the brain.*

vii. *Apex Energetics – Neuro-Flam (K-46) is a phenol-flavonoid complex designed to specifically target brain health as it relates to microglial activity in the brain-immune system.*

viii. *Apex Energetics - Metacrin-DX (K-10) is a formula designed to support phase 1 and phase 2 detoxication.*

 ix. Apex Energetics – GlutenFlam (k-52) is a one-of-a-kind digestive aid that features powerful digestive enzymes to address unintended gluten and casein exposure.

Keep in mind that if you drop a pebble in the water, the greatest impact is the ripple directly next to the surface of the water where the pebble made contact. The same is true with stimulating neural pathways. However, there's always a ripple effect which flows out to benefit more systems in the body that you may be initially trying to help. When you think about stimulating the neural pathways, the more that you can fire at a time, the greater the positive effects that come from that stimulation. The following exercises will help you "fire" the Vagus nerve and keep it active and healthy.

 4. At-home Vagus Nerve Stimulation Exercises

Gargling: Gargle for two minutes straight, and I mean gargle like your life depends on it. To accentuate the effect of this stimulation, try fixating on a certain point or part of the wall that's above you. To multiply the positive effects of this even more, do these two things while also doing non-linear complex movements like writing out your name in "air letters" with your free hand or spelling your first and last name.

Ear Lobes: Massaging your outer ear lobes stimulates the Vagus nerve.

The "No No" Exercise: As you focus your attention on a point on the wall, put your feet together and fixate on that point while also rotating your head from right to left *and* humming the "Happy Birthday" song. Then change the exercise by moving your head back and forth as if you're saying "yes yes."

Humming: Humming seems to activate very beneficial parts of the brain that are connected to the Vagus nerve and therefore essential to your gut health.

Gagging: If you're brave enough, try gagging yourself approximately three times until you tear up. Sound intense? It is, but it's one of the best ways to stimulate the Vagus nerve.

If you start to implement these changes, you may begin to notice decreased bloating, gas and diarrhea. You'll notice less brain fog and enjoy improved gut function. We need to see our gut and brain as one because they directly communicate with one another. Now that we've covered your gut, let's move to the next key to solving chronic health problems.

SHARED FOLLOW THROUGH

CHAPTER 12

HOW EXAMS HELP YOU HEAL

WHAT IS AN EXAM?

In our clinic, every patient's journey begins with a thorough functional neurological exam. This is a head-to-toe neurological evaluation on you. We do this because we treat every single person as a unique, one-of-a-kind case. Think of the way a detective picks up the trail of a murder case that's gone cold. That's how we approach each person's tangled web of dysfunction. The exam is like cracking open that file and looking at every piece of evidence in a new light.

Many times, exams are used more as a "check off" list for doctors. They're such a rich opportunity for the doctor to gather valuable data about their patient, yet they don't bother to ask enough questions or get the right kind of data needed to really solve the patient's problems. Too often, doctors come in with preconceived notions and they don't put their hands on their patients. Yes, you actually have to touch your patient to do a neurological exam.

In my experience, performing a thorough neurological exam is both an art and a science. The art aspect focuses on how to perform the exam fluidly and in a systematic way that identifies which systems are not functioning properly and are likely damaged. It's also an art form to identify and then assist the most devastated areas of the patient's brain. The science portion comes from all the neurology in classroom learning at the universities as well as textbooks. Most doctors can do the science part. It's the art part that's rare.

I use the same acronym to guide me through every single patient exam, and it's called POPQRST.

> P - Primary complaint. What health issue is having the biggest negative impact on their life? Has anyone else in their family had this issue before?

> O - Onset. When did the symptoms start? And is the primary complaint staying the same or getting worse?

> P - Pain. What provokes the pain and what makes it better?

> Q - Quality of pain. Is there burning, numbness, or tingling?

> R - Radiate. Does the pain radiate out or does it stay local?

> S - Severity. Rank the pain on a scale of 1-10. How bad is it?

> T - Time. What time of day or night is the primary complaint worse?

During this exam, we also test the patient's oxygen levels to determine if they're anemic or not. The body can't heal unless it has the proper supply of oxygen, so this is a crucial first step. We also take their blood pressure (which gives us another hint about their oxygen levels), have their blood drawn and perform intensive blood work, and do glucose testing. All of these tests are getting baseline measurements on the patient's seven keys to health because these keys provide the clues I use to untangle their web of dysfunction and heal their chronic health problems.

During the neurological testing portion of the exam, I use a tuning fork to test the sensitivity of their nervous system. I take the tuning fork, place it on their sternum, and allow them to feel the vibration. That vibration represents a value of 10 and serves as our reference point. Then, I do the same thing but put the tuning fork against their big toe, their thumbs and their shoulders.

Next, I do a two-point discrimination test where I make sure the radial nerve (the nerve which controls sensation in the back of the arm and forearm) is intact and functioning. Then, I test the lower extremities using a two point discrimination test. I check the L-4 saphenous nerve (controls sensation to the inside of the lower leg) and L-5 superficial peroneal nerve (controls the outside of the lower leg). I follow that test with the digit span test where I evaluate the Median nerve which controls the thumb and first and second fingers. I then check Ulnar nerve sensation to part of the ring finger and little finger. Next, I perform the digit span test on the toes via the L-5 superficial peroneal nerve which controls all sensation on the top of the feet as well as all toes (except the small toe which is controlled by the S-1 sural nerve). These tests give me a good indication of how the patient's peripheral nervous system as well as the parietal lobe, located in the back half of the brain, is functioning. Next, I test their reflexes which tells me how well their motor reflexes are responding. Human beings have 10 motor reflexes, and I test all reflexes to see how well their cerebellum, brain and spinal cord are working.

CEREBELLUM TESTS:

After that, I ask them to stand up, if they can, and put their feet together and close their eyes. Next, I'll ask the patient to close their eyes and put their right foot in front of the left foot. Then, I have them switch legs. I follow that exercise up by asking them to alternately lift each leg off the ground and hold it at a 90 degree angle. If your cerebellum is functioning optimally you should be able to maintain each balance/stability test for fifteen seconds. I continue the neurological part of the exam by testing them for smell, fine motor skills, and many more factors that show me the state of their neurological health.

Finger to nose test: I ask the patient to close their eyes and try to place their little finger on the tip of their nose. Fingertip to nose tip. If they miss, they probably have a decreased functioning cerebellum on the side being tested.

It's important to approach an exam with humility and curiosity because I'm working in the field of probabilities, not absolutes. If you're aspiring to be an accountant or an engineer and seeking absolute answers, this probably is not the field for you. Practically nothing in neurology is absolute. Approaching the patient as if they're a completely new, one-of-a-kind case is the most important mental shift I make every time I prepare to do an exam.

THE FUNDAMENTALS OF AN EFFECTIVE EXAM

When a patient comes into the clinic for an exam, they'll have already filled out their paperwork and we have their blood work results on hand. I start the exam by asking them some questions. Then I move into the primary pillars of executing a great exam.

Pillar One: Where is the problem? Is it neurological, metabolic or both?

Pillar Two: How much can we stimulate the system before it fatigues?

Pillar Three: Do I think I can improve this patient's well being?

Often, the exam reveals new and insightful information that helps us "crack the case." One of my favorite stories is of a young lady who came into the clinic for an exam. She was twenty-one years old and had been a soccer player before her condition forced her to quit sports. She was afflicted with terrible migraine headaches on nearly a daily basis. She had seen multiple medical doctors including neurologists and had all traditional healthcare testing performed. Any kind of major stimulation or specific indoor lighting sent her into a severe pain. If she got out of the car and the sun hit her eyes wrong, she started having migraines.

Through neurological testing and the exam, I discovered she had a possible autoimmune disorder, and her oxygen levels were very low. Her feet and hands were also very cold which meant they weren't getting adequate oxygen. It turned out she had developed autoimmunity against her gut.

I prescribed a treatment plan of Vagal nerve stimulation, the 10-week brain and body detox program, brain stimulation therapy, Trigenics nerve, muscle and joint therapy for her neck, ears, sinuses and jaw, along with many other home-based modalities. Once we identified the root cause of her problem, which was the autoimmune condition, we began this treatment protocol that targeted the cause of her dysfunction. Within four months, she no longer had any migraines. Since then, she is back playing soccer and wants to become a physical therapist. This is the power of doing the right kind of exam. The clues I found in the neurological exam helped me figure out what part of the body was malfunctioning, and when we addressed the root of the problem, she got her life back.

Another favorite story is of a patient who had been told he needed to move to an assisted living facility because of his poor health and lack of coordination. He initially came in for "frozen" shoulders that wouldn't allow him to move his arms above 90 degrees. Through a neurological exam, we discovered the part of the brain that was malfunctioning. We used brain stimulation therapy to activate certain muscle groups to reset the neurological receptors in that part of the body, which allowed the brain to recognize and execute the full range of motion. Within four minutes of his first treatment, he went from being able to lift his arms and hands to only as high as his shoulder height, to lifting them above his head, full range of motion of 180 degrees. From that point, we worked together to heal a whole cascade of chronic health problems that were holding him back and limiting his quality of life. Within nine months of receiving treatment at our clinic, he and his family were back to adventuring the Appalachian Trail. They've since traveled to national parks out west."

This is why I treat every single person as a unique, one-of-a-kind case. Every person's tangled web of dysfunction is different and caused by a different combination of dysfunctional processes. The exam is how we open that cold-case file and start to uncover what's going on beneath the surface.

CHAPTER 13

OUR PROGRAM

THE PHASES OF DECLINE

The "phases of decline" refer to the stages someone struggling with chronic health problems will experience as their dysfunctional process advances. While this book is ultimately about hope and the encouragement that it is often possible to stop and reverse physical damage and disorders, you also need to take these phases of decline seriously because there is a point of no return. At this point, the body becomes so damaged that it's not possible to regenerate your health to a normal state. Let's take a look at the phases of decline for the three most common maladies I see in my clinic—brain disorders, knee pain, and neuropathy.

PHASES OF DECLINE FOR BRAIN DISORDERS

Phase One: Full Health

No symptoms expressed at all.

Phase Two: Easily Dismissible Symptoms

These are things like brain fog that just won't go away, difficulty focusing and concentrating for long periods of time, and a loss of attention to the things you normally enjoy and love. At this point, your brain cells are actually dying, yet most people won't take action, instead choosing to casually dismiss the changes. The patient usually doesn't take responsibility or action, at least not yet.

Phase Three/Four: Recognizable Symptoms

At this stage, things are beginning to progress. You may walk into a room and forget why you walked in there in the first place. Or you may call someone on the phone and forget why you called them. This is an advanced stage of brain degeneration. This is the point where the adult kids may tease their parents about having "old timers" syndrome or say things like "Mom is just losing it…" At this stage, it's very important to filter who you listen to. Your healthcare provider, your kids, your friends, or your spouse may laugh it off, but it's nothing to joke about. At this phase, you must stand up and take responsibility for your health. If you know something isn't right, keep pursuing a solution until you get answers.

Phase Five: The Limitation of Matter

At this stage, the brain is degenerated to the point where the person is no longer motivated and simply doesn't have the brain ability to solve their own problems. They no longer see themselves as the problem; instead, everyone else has a problem. When someone reaches this stage, it is very hard and nearly impossible to bring them back. It's a very serious case when someone gets to this stage. It's called "limitation of matter" because at this point, the brain has degenerated so far that it's unable to regenerate and repair to its former state. I don't accept patients for care who are at this stage of degeneration.

Common Treatments for Brain Disorders:

These are the common in-clinic treatments that I do for brain-based disorders.

- Clear Mind neurofeedback program - this tool instantly and non-invasively identifies brain dysfunction. I use these results to know which areas of the brain to stimulate to help it begin functioning optimally again.

- Exercise with oxygen therapy - This is simply putting an oxygen mask on the patient and having them complete a low impact exercise while breathing in pure oxygen.

- Hako-Med - This powerful machine helps stimulate proper nerve function.

- Pulse Electro-Magnetic Field (PEMF) machine - This machine is like a battery re-charger for your body. It helps to recharge the cells of the body to the perfect charge to maintain optimal cellular function.

- At-Home Exercises - Vagal stimulation exercises, 10-week brain and body detox, and proper nutritional supplementation.

PHASES OF DECLINE FOR KNEE PAIN

I classify chronic knee pain as anything that has existed for three months or longer. Most of the people who come see me for knee pain have had it for years, if not decades, and can barely walk or get out of a chair. They often have difficulty getting out of bed or off the couch, and their life is severely impacted by their pain. One of the first things I do with every knee pain patient is take x-rays of the knee. We can use regenerative medicine at the clinic, but in order for that treatment to be effective, there has to be a space between the knee joint as seen on the radiograph. The space is important because it means there is still tissue present that can be rehabilitated. If there's no space, they've reached the limitation of matter and have to be referred out for a knee replacement. I don't accept everyone that comes into the office as a patient. If I do the exam and, based on their results, I don't think I can help them, I refer the patient to a health professional who can better assist them.

However, if the x-ray shows enough spacing in the joint, I may start with a regenerative medicine treatment plan to help them eliminate their chronic pain and regain mobility. Here are some of the solutions that have worked exceptionally well for our knee pain patients.

Common Treatments for Knee Pain:

- Knee Decompression - This is a machine that decompresses the knee and opens up the joint space, promoting healing and pain relief.

- Oxygen therapy with exercise - I talked about this treatment earlier in the book, but this is simply putting an oxygen mask on the patient and having them complete a low impact exercise while breathing in oxygen.

- Hako-Med - This powerful machine helps stimulate proper nerve function.

- Laser therapy - This treatment decreases inflammation and pain by dilating the capillaries to promote blood flow and encourage the healing properties to access the joint.

- Pulse Electro-Magnetic Field (PEMF) machine - This machine is like a battery re-charger for your body. It helps to recharge the cells of the body to the perfect charge to maintain optimal cellular function.

- Trigenics - This modality activates the two main receptors of the brain so that they fire into the cerebellum, spinal cord and brain to decrease pain, increase mobility and increase strength.

PHASES OF DECLINE FOR NEUROPATHY:

Neuropathy patients are usually the most complicated cases because neuropathy can be caused by so many different dysfunctions. These patients often have oxygen problems, glucose problems, and their brain has deteriorated because of a lack of stimulation from their feet. Many people with neuropathy also have erectile or sexual dysfunction.

Phase One: The feet begin tingling or experiencing a pins and needles sensation.

Phase Two: Coldness and color changes in the toes and feet.

Phase Three: The tingling becomes a burning pain.

Phase Four: Loss of sensation in the legs, feet, toes.

Common Treatments for Neuropathy:

- Blood sugar regulation - I work with the patient to help them balance their blood sugar so their neurological system can stabilize and begin the work of healing.

- Spinal decompression - Many patients with neuropathy have L5 damage so I use decompression therapy to relieve the pressure on that area of the spine.

- Oxygen therapy with exercise - I talked about this treatment earlier in the book, but this is simply putting an oxygen mask on the patient and having them complete a low impact exercise while breathing in oxygen.

- Hako-Med on their feet - This powerful machine helps stimulate proper nerve function.

- Laser therapy - This treatment decreases inflammation and pain by dilating the capillaries to promote blood flow and encourage the healing properties to access the joint.

- Pulse Electro-Magnetic Field (PEMF) machine - This machine is like a battery re-charger for your body. It helps to recharge the cells of the body to the perfect charge to maintain optimal cellular function.

- Trigenics - This modality activates the two main receptors of the brain so that they fire into the cerebellum, spinal cord and brain to decrease pain and increase mobility.

- Clear Mind neurofeedback program - this tool instantly and non-invasively identifies brain dysfunction. I use these results to know which areas of the brain to stimulate to help it start functioning optimally again.

- At-Home Exercises - Brain-Body-Gut 10-week detox and proper nutritional supplementation.

CUSTOM MADE

A truly custom, one-of-a-kind healthcare program will impact your health in a way you've never experienced before because it is created uniquely for you. I don't accept everyone for care. If someone isn't fully committed, they're too neurologically damaged, or they're too far degenerated, I'm not going to take them for care and waste their time or money. When I accept someone for care, I make them a promise that I'm on this journey with them, and we're in it to win it. I will exhaust every option I know in order to optimize their recovery. However, we both need to have realistic expectations. If their expectations are beyond what I can give them, we need to realign. I'm always going to under promise and over deliver, and sometimes tough love requires telling people the truth that they don't want to hear.

A custom healthcare program to heal your chronic disease always comes as a result of a thorough and effective neurological examination process, and it always addresses all aspects of your metabolic and neurological health. However, the truth is that if they don't follow the program I prescribe them, they're probably not going to get the results they want. No one is going to care more about your health than you. If you don't want to be well, live vibrantly, and leave a legacy, no one is going to do it for you. I'm totally committed to the patient, but they need to be "all in" too.

CHAPTER 14

TAKING THE NEXT STEP TOWARD HEALING

Congratulations—you've made it to the final chapter! You've learned a lot about your body and the differences between traditional medicine and how a dedicated chiropractic functional neurology practitioner like me works with their patients. So, how do you know when you're ready to take that next step and make your first appointment? And when do you know you've found the right doctor for you?

By choosing to work with me, you are opening the door to a different way of doing things. You shouldn't take your decision lightly. Just as it is with medical doctors, chiropractic health practitioners vary greatly in their areas of specialization, approach to treatment options, cutting edge diagnostic tools and treatment technologies. We are going to spend a lot of time together initially, so we will want to ensure it's a good fit for you and your condition before you commit. Because the healing process involves your active participation, I'm sharing my ideas on the ideal doctor/patient relationship that you can use as a guide to making sure you're ready to take your next steps.

YOU ARE OPEN TO A DIFFERENT WAY OF HEALING

Maybe you feel like you have been painted into a corner saying, "I don't want to go in that direction. I don't want to end up like so and so. I've had surgery, and I don't want to go through that again."

Each year I see hundreds of patients suffering from what they believe are permanent conditions. They've been told by their traditional healthcare practitioner that nothing can be done and they have to "learn to live with it." They keep taking the multitudes of medications that have been prescribed to them and see no improvement as their condition slowly worsens over time. I'm here to tell you that is not necessarily true.

Maybe you've been told by your medical doctor that there's no hope for you. Your health, and therefore your life, CAN change for the better. The first step toward healing is understanding that your future is in your hands and no one else's. Your health can change, but you have to first decide to want to make that change. Your life, your purpose, and all you have to offer are too important to be held back by chronic health problems. Please recognize that while you may have been led to believe it is impossible to change your current course of health, you must open your mind to an alternative approach with a new way of thinking and method to healing. It is then that new possibilities, hope and a feeling of optimism toward healing can become your reality.

The only thing stopping you from going from where you are to where you wish you could be is what you're not willing to do. You need to ask if you are the limiting factor. Do you want to be passive (drugs or surgery) in your health care? Or do you want to be active in learning and doing the things that will get to the root causes of your condition and maintain your progress over time? If you're the latter, oftentimes I can help you reach your personal goals.

YOU'RE WILLING TO ENTER A PARTNERSHIP.

Did you ever hear that saying that if you keep doing what you're doing, you'll keep getting what you're getting? Are you at the point where it feels like your situation is as good as it gets? And although you aren't happy with your circumstances, do you feel like you're out of options?

Are you willing to engage in a different kind of doctor/patient relationship than you're used to so you can finally get the results you deserve?

What I am saying here is that this is a partnership. You must first take responsibility for your current condition. Yes, I understand you may have listened to other doctors and it just didn't get you to where you wanted to be. It's all water under the bridge. We can only change what we do going forward. It may be a departure from what you've believed or done in the past, but you have an opportunity to own your role and trust in the process of being an active participant in care. Once we establish that trust and belief, I will do everything in my power to help you optimize your recovery. It's about leading you down the road to regaining the lifestyle you so deserve.

Are you ready to commit to better health by working toward goals? Are you so tired of being tired that you'll do whatever it takes to feel better, even when it gets hard? When a prospective patient is dedicated to putting in the work, doctors like me are excited to share their wisdom and begin walking beside you on your path to better health.

YOU HAVE TO CARE ABOUT YOUR HEALTH MORE THAN ANYONE ELSE DOES

I want to be able to help each and every person who walks through our door. Everyone at our clinic feels compelled to help you reach your goals and expects that you are just as vested in the results as we are. Actually, you should be vested even more. After all, this is your life we're talking about. Nobody can care more about your health than you can.

It's important for you to understand your motivation. When you know that you're working toward your "why," it will keep you moving in the right direction, even when things may become difficult.

Your "why" can be simple. Maybe you want to be able to sit in the stands to watch a grandchild play baseball. You want to walk around the block with your spouse, travel, or take a cruise with your family.

When you have a clear picture of what you're working toward, and you can tie it to doing it for yourself and someone else, you can share your goals and have them help you stay accountable for achieving them.

I've asked many patients over the years what joy, happiness, peace of mind or sense of security for the future is their condition stealing from their life. Often, they'll tell me they aren't worried as much about themselves but are concerned they won't be able to continue their independence of living on their own and have started to become too dependent on family members for help. They feel like they are becoming a burden to them. This becomes their motivation or "why".

WHAT IS THE TYPICAL INITIAL PROCESS WHEN WORKING WITH OUR CLINIC?

Your reasons for wanting to feel better are personal, and we take our jobs personally as well. Healing can be an exciting process when you decide to go all in and commit to taking an active role on your journey to feeling better. As you've read, working with a practitioner like me is different than what you've experienced with your traditional medical doctors during those appointments.

As your healthcare professional, our goals are always about you, not us. And no, we're not here just to crack your back. It's about restoring your lifestyle and getting you back to doing the things you want to be doing again. Making that first appointment is a big step. It's a commitment to taking back your life, and not to be taken lightly.

After going through your initial screening, I will sit down with you and simply have a conversation. We'll discuss your answers to all the questions. What's bringing you in to the clinic? Where are you having the problem? How did it happen? When does it happen? Did you have any history of injuries or trauma? What have you tried in the past to help your condition? What do you want to be able to do? What is your "why?" This discussion typically isn't as much about your pain as it is about what you want to be able to do daily and on a long-term basis without difficulty.

Together, we'll take everything into account—from a neurological standpoint to your range of motion, your strength and even imaging and bloodwork. Once all of that information is gathered and discussed, you'll learn more about the forms of treatment that will benefit you the most along with an action plan. Typically, you'll be in the clinic several days a week at the beginning of your care and taper that off over time as you improve.

Remember, you are ultimately in charge of your health and wellness in this lifetime.

If you'd like to learn more about my practice, visit HarrisburgWellnessCenter.com or call 704-455-2211.

I look forward to helping you see what's possible when you think outside of the box!

ABOUT THE AUTHOR

Dr. Segarra is a 1998 graduate of the National University of Health Sciences in Chicago, Illinois. He has practiced in the state of North Carolina ever since. He has treated more than 20,000 patients. He is certified in functional neurology, spinal and knee decompression, treating extremity conditions, Webster Pregnancy, Trigenics, Instrument Assisted Soft Tissue Mobilization (IASTM or Scraping), Activator and ProAdjuster techniques. He has served as a board member of the Southwest Cabarrus Rotary Club and has organized and run local meetings for the Cabarrus Chamber of Commerce.

Prior to attaining his doctorate of chiropractic, Dr. Segarra earned both a B.A. degree from the State University of New York at Binghamton in Biology and a B.S. degree from the National University of Health Sciences in Human Biology. While at Binghamton, he served as an athletic trainer giving him the knowledge and ability to diagnose and treat many sports related injuries more effectively.

Dr. Segarra is a unique chiropractor to this area. His experience working at First Choice Family Healthcare in Raleigh, Chicago's Edgewater Hospital and the Chicago AIDS Alternative Health Project provides for a training few chiropractors have. In each setting he worked in collaboration with other healthcare professionals including medical doctors, physical therapists, exercise physiologists, psychologists, acupuncturists and massage therapists.

A team approach was utilized in addressing and treating each individual patient's needs. He has found working in unison with other healthcare providers yields maximum results and better patient outcomes. This networking and team approach is a concept he brings to Harrisburg and the Charlotte, NC area.

Most importantly, Dr. Segarra, wants you to know that he cares about your health and wishes to bring a higher quality of life to the community, one patient at a time.

Outside of the clinic he loves spending time with his wife, Colleen, and four children: Jack, Lucy, Seth and Ethan along with their dog and cat. Dr. Segarra is very active in his children's sports and activities which include baseball, basketball, golf and swimming. Every member of the family is active and gets adjusted regularly. All of his kids have been receiving chiropractic treatments since birth. In Dr. Segarra's spare time he enjoys golfing, sports games, reading books, coaching and attending his kids' sporting events. He is also active with their elementary school's "Be There Dad" chapter and serves as a mentor for students in need.